AGHOAGNI GOUAJIO GILLES GAEL

VALUE OF DEXAMETHASONE IN THE PREVENTION OF NAUSEA AND VOMITING

AGHOAGNI GOUAJIO GILLES GAEL

VALUE OF DEXAMETHASONE IN THE PREVENTION OF NAUSEA AND VOMITING

ScienciaScripts

Imprint

Any brand names and product names mentioned in this book are subject to trademark, brand or patent protection and are trademarks or registered trademarks of their respective holders. The use of brand names, product names, common names, trade names, product descriptions etc. even without a particular marking in this work is in no way to be construed to mean that such names may be regarded as unrestricted in respect of trademark and brand protection legislation and could thus be used by anyone.

Cover image: www.ingimage.com

This book is a translation from the original published under ISBN 978-3-8417-7830-7.

Publisher:
Sciencia Scripts
is a trademark of
Dodo Books Indian Ocean Ltd. and OmniScriptum S.R.L publishing group

120 High Road, East Finchley, London, N2 9ED, United Kingdom
Str. Armeneasca 28/1, office 1, Chisinau MD-2012, Republic of Moldova, Europe
Printed at: see last page
ISBN: 978-620-5-83937-9

Copyright © AGHOAGNI GOUAJIO GILLES GAEL
Copyright © 2023 Dodo Books Indian Ocean Ltd. and OmniScriptum S.R.L publishing group

Contents

To the Lord GOD

The almighty creator of heaven and earth. The one without whom this work could not have been done. I thank you and glorify you on this day for the breath of life, health and peace that you give to me and to all my loved ones every day.

Thank you for allowing me to obtain this degree. Grant that I may always live by your word and never be turned away from your face. Give me the power to

to spread around me this love that you have freely given us and that I may

and may I always glorify you in the practice of medicine.

Thank you

DEDICATED

> To my father Mr. AGHOAGNI Jean Marie. Dad, I thank you for the love you have for me. You have always believed in me and have always made sure that I lack nothing. You have always encouraged and galvanized me so that I could always give the best of myself. You taught us discipline, respect, love of work and of each other and instilled family spirit. Thank you for all the sacrifices you have made on my behalf. I dedicate this diploma to you as a token of my appreciation and I hope to do you honour. May the Lord grant you health and longevity so that we can enjoy the fruits of this work. I love you.

> To my mother Mrs AGHOAGNI Melanie. I can't find the right words to tell you how I feel about you. Thank you for all the sacrifices you made for me and for the whole family. You always wanted me to be free from want. This work is yours because the person I am today is the fruit of your labour, your sacrifices and your prayers. You knew how to trust me at an early age and instil moral and spiritual values in me. I am proud to be your child and I hope that on this day I also make you proud. I love you.

> To Mother Ernestine. Thank you for your encouragement and support. I thank you for the family spirit that you have brought and maintained within the family. May we always live in this peace as long as GOD grants us the breath of life.

> To my little brothers and sisters (**Merline, Arlette, Nelson and Joël**). I thank you for your affection, your encouragement and your prayers. May the Lord always strengthen this brotherly love and understanding between us. I hope that this result will serve as an example to you and that you will dare to do better than I did.

> **my late grandmother Mama TSAGUE Teclaire**. Thank you for the good times spent by your side because you were always tender and affectionate towards me and all your family whatever the circumstances. With you I was always serene because I counted on your love and your prayers which undoubtedly helped us and which accompany us until now because I know that

where you are you will always continue to intercede with the Lord for your family. Thank you for everything. May the land of our ancestors be light to you. Rest in peace.

ACKNOWLEDGEMENTS

> To Mali and all its people. Thank you for your welcome and your hospitality. Our stay was pleasant.

> To the faculty of the Faculty of Medicine and Odonto-stomatology. Thank you for the quality of the courses given.

> To Professor DIALLO Abdoulaye. We have been marked by the conviviality, the human warmth, and the simplicity that characterize you. Thank you for all the teachings and advice given to us.

> To Professor DIANGO DJIBO Mahamane You have amazed us with your eloquence and your intellectual culture. We have been able to count on a man of value, both medically and humanly, concerned with research, knowledge and work well done. We thank you for this.

> To Dr. Broulaye SAMAKE, thank you for your scientific rigour. Thanks to you we have developed a critical and scientific mind. Thank you for your advice. May God bless you.

> To my grandmothers MEDONNANG Pauline and FEUJIO Christine. Thank you for your encouragement and your prayers. Thank you for always thinking of me. May GOD grant you many more years on earth, health and peace of mind.

> To my aunt Dr MBADUET Yvonne married to Dr WAMBA. Thank you for your encouragement and your support that you always brought me at the right time. May God bless you and all your family.

> To mother Honorine epouse TCHOUPA. I thank you for all the sacrifices made for me since my birth. May GOD grant you health and happiness in your home.

> To my aunts Dr MAAKENG Cecilia epouse Maitre NANFAH, mother Jeanne d'Arc KAGHO, mother Irene NGOUADJIO, my mother Clarisse KEMGOU, mother Marie TSOPBOU, mother Virginie KAZE, mother GNIZEKO Helene. Thank you for your prayers, your encouragement and your advice. May God grant you longevity and health.

> To my uncles: Papa TEMGOUA Andre, Papa Jean Marie TSOPONANG,

Uncle Denis. Thank you for your advice, your encouragement and your support.

> To all the NGOUADJIO family. Thank you for your prayers and your encouragement; for the cohesion, the understanding and the good living which reign in all the houses.

> To the whole TEKA family. Thank you for your encouragement and support. May the Lord allow us to be united and remain so throughout our time on earth.

> To my great sister and my great brothers: DONFACK Desta, KAZE Duplex, ADEPI Aristhide, ANOUAZI Ebeny. I have learned a lot and fully blossomed with you and it is thanks to you that I have been able to develop this scientific spirit that animates me. May God always fill us with grace and grant us a long life.

> To Dr NANFAH Patricia epouse POUFONG "my mother" from Bamako. I thank you for all that you have done for me. You allowed me to come to Mali, you welcomed me and always took care of me during all your stay in Mali while still a student. May God fill you with grace.

> To the A.E.E.S.C.M (Association of Cameroonian Students and Trainees in Mali). Thank you because in your bosom I discovered myself and blossomed. Thank you to the members of the promotions (ASTRA, SARTRE, SEGALEN, PRADIER, CESAR, SPARTE, ASTURIE, STATE, TROIE, ROME, PARIS, ALSACE)

> My friends in Bamako: Dr SONFACK Pamela, Dr KAMDEM Lolitha, Dr Thierry Martial, Dr TCHOMCHOUA Stephane, Dr MBASSI Cedric, Dr NEMSI

Int^ret de la dexaméthasone dans la prevention des NVPO en chirurgie ORL Daniel, Dr MODI Yannick, Dr Cheick DIOUF, Dr TCHOGANG Nina, Dr KENFACK Hermann, Dr TIOKENG Rodrigue, Dr PESSEU Lucrece, Dr NGADJEU Francis, Dr Armand KAMKUMO, Dr YEPGUE Guy, Dr FAMO Roch. Thank you for everything because you guided me and gave me advice so that I could adapt to the conditions of life in Bamako and that I could flourish. > To my family in Bamako, the TCHOMCHOUA-MODI family:

> My brothers and sisters (Cyril MBASSI, Gregory NGASSA, Dr MANI Danielle, Dr FOTSO Michelle, Natacha MBEUMO "my twin"). Thank you for the fraternal spirit that you have created in this family;

> my sons and daughters (Martial FASSEU, Hermann NGALEU, Yannick MBIA, Kevin KAMSU, Simplice DJOMZO ,Ornella TCHANQUE, Stephanie NGUEMA,Missa KAMISSOKO, Floribert FOTSO, Nadine NDEFRE, Yvette NGOMO, Manuella TCHAPDA, Armel TCHOMTCHOUA, Rodrigue BANGTE, Stephane OWONA, Yvan ATANGANA, C. Damien TCHUISSEU, KUATE Fabrice, Lynda SAMO, Yvette NGUEAGNI, Rachel DZUIWOUO , Richie TCHUISI , Cindy WEMBE, Pavel NGUEKENG). You all accepted me as the "father" of this great family after the initiators left. It was an honour and a good experience for me. We had good and bad moments but despite that we remained united. To the young people I urge you to work hard because success comes with effort. Thank you for all

> To the promotion of Pr ASSA SIDIBE. Thank you for all the moments shared together.

> To the DEGAULLE promotion. Just saying that word brings tears to my eyes. I could only belong to this class. We shared unforgettable moments and I am proud of it. I have grown and matured in this class. I hope that this family spirit will last even after Bamako. Gaullois and Gaulloises, I love you.

> To YMELE NANA Cedric. We met in Bamako but we understood each other very quickly and you were always there whenever I needed your help. I don't doubt your friendship and I know that it is reciprocal. You are the "twin and friend" I never had. Thank you for your support in times of trouble and joy. THANK YOU.

> A MOLO BIETEKE A. Ines. Thank you for all the good times we had together. It's true that we had some misunderstandings but I know that I can count on your unconditional friendship and vice versa. May God bless you and fill you with grace.

> To MANEMEZA MBEUMO Natacha "my twin". Thank you for all the good moments shared together, whether during the "boss" periods with the stress and your tears, or during the training courses and the moments of atmosphere with your simplicity and your joy of living. You are special.

> To KOUENKAM NANA Manuella. Thank you for your advice and friendship. I pray that you can remain open and sociable as you have been lately.

> To NGUEAGNI Yvette (my daughter from Bamako) thank you for the support, encouragement and special affection you gave me. You always cared about me, my health and what I was going to eat. Thank you for everything.

> To NGALEU Hermann. Thank you for your friendship because you are like a brother to me. You understand me and very often I have had to rely on your help which you have always given me for free. Thank you and bless you.

> To my study group: Dr WOKDEN Sonia, Dr FOMO Doryne, Fabrice KEMBOU, GUEMNING Viviane. It was a pleasure to share this experience with you. All these moments of galere, stress and "boss" lived together are unforgettable moments. Thank you for your encouragement and your advice. Be blessed.

> To my friends: Wilson NJAKOU, Jean Jacques AKOUA, Dr Leonel TCHAMO, NANA Manuella, Natacha MBEUMO, Dr FOMO Doryne, Dr WOKDEN Sonia, Leattitia TCHAWA, CHAWA Adhemar, Dr OMOCK Sandrine, Alida MEZEUBOU, Arnold SIMO, Yvan NOGUIA, Dr LISSOH Patricia. Thank you for accepting me as a friend with all my faults and for giving me your help when I needed it. May God bless you.

> To TEKA Lydie (sister) and LATAGUIA Flaure. Thank you for the unconditional love and esteem you have for me. I hope I can always return it to you. Thank you for all

> To all my neighbours: Dr AWOMO Rosine, NGALEU Hermann "ramos", EKOUNE Michel, SOUMANI Steve, TATSITSA Yannick, Dr Leonel AMOUSSOU, Mylaine DONFACK, NITCHEU Joelle, NGUEAGNI Yvette, Sophie DEGUENON, Daouda, Fortune, Prudence OMAM, Idriss, Dr Eleazar

DAO, Barou SOGOBA, Elysee. Thank you for your encouragement and support. It was a pleasure to have you as neighbours if not co-tenants as we are well in the only courtyard where everyone feels at home in any room. Please keep up the spirit of brotherhood.

> To the staff of the DARMU (Department of Anaesthesia, Intensive Care and Emergency Medicine) of the Gabriel Toure University Hospital. Thank you for your welcome and your adoption because with you I always felt welcome as well as with the chiefs and elders (Pr Abdoulaye DIALLO, Pr Djibo DIANGO, Dr Broulaye SAMAKE, Dr MANGANE, Dr MAIGA H., Dr TOGOLA, Dr KEITA B., Dr KASSOUGUE A. Dr TOURE , Dr DIARRA D.,Dr DAO , Dr JEAN de DIEU, major DIABATE, Marie Cecile, Dr Binta DIALLO, Mme SY, ...), the interns (Lamine TRAORE, Hermann NOUBISSIE, Natacha MBEUMO, Aoua DOUMBIA , Allassane DOUMBIA, Emma NSIA, Wilson NJAKOU, Lynda MONTHEU, Alida MEZEUBOU, SANOGO, Bongana MAIGA, YOAN, NANA

Int^ret of dexaméthasone in the prevention of PONV in ENT surgery Manuella) that with all the nursing teams(Baga , Moussa Berthe, Soumaila , Josue, ...).

>   To the staff of the ENT-CCF department. Thank you for your welcome and your collaboration.

>   To my team on duty: Aoua DOUMBIA , TOGOLA, DEMBELE, Mariam DAGNOGO, Pamela SAMIZA , Fatoumata SAMAKE, Binta SIDIBE ,Fatoumata SIDIBE, SANGARE. Thank you for all the support you have given me to be able to lead this team. I was very happy to work with you and I hope that you will keep this dynamic and scientific spirit that you have in you.

>   To my cousins: Leopold MAAKENG, MEZANOU Huguette, Merlin KAGHO, KAZE Charly, Manuella NANFAH, . Thank you for your support which has done me a lot of good. May the Lord bless you.

>   To my friends from high school (TEFONOU Igor, TCHONTA Isabelle, LIENOU Thierry, Dr CHEUYEM Zobel). Thank you for your moral support.

>   To all those whose names do not appear and who, in one way or another,

have supported me and contributed to the elaboration of this work, I thank you and may God bless you.

TO OUR MASTER AND PRESIDENT OF THE JURY
Professor SAMBA KARIM TIMBO:
> **Lecturer in ENT and CCF;**
> **Founding member and secretary general of the Malian ENT Society;**
> **Member of the Faculty Assembly of the WFOS;**
> **Member of the Ivorian ENT Society;**
> **Member of the ENT Society of French-speaking Africa (SORLAF);**
> **Member of the Portmann Institute;**
> **Head of the DER of Surgery ;**
> **Medical Director at the Gabriel Toure University Hospital;**

Dear Master,

The spontaneity with which you agreed to chair this jury is a testimony to the immense honour you have bestowed on us and to your attachment to scientific work. Your kindness and your open-mindedness, which are equalled only by your rigour and your sense of effort in your work, have confirmed our admiration for you.

Please accept, dear master, the sincere expression of our deepest respect.

TO OUR MASTER AND JUDGE

DOCTOR MAMADOU KARIM TOURE

> **Anesthesiologist-resuscitator, specialist in:**

> **Emergency and disaster medicine;**

> **Neuroanesthesia-resuscitation;**

> **Maternal, neonatal and infant resuscitation anaesthesia;**

> **Oncology anaesthesia, pain management and palliative care;**

> **Hospital practitioner ;**

> **Head of the anaesthesia and emergency department of the Centre**

Hospitalier Mere Enfant le LUXEMBOURG (CHME) ;

> **Member of SARMU-MALI;**

> **Member of SARANF.**

Dear Master,

You are doing us a great honour by accepting to take part in this jury.

We cannot thank you enough for your participation in perfecting this work. We have been marked by your courtesy, humility and availability to us.

Please find here, dear Master, the testimony of our deep gratitude.

TO OUR MASTER AND JUDGE

DOCTOR SIAKA SOUMAORO

> **Specialist in ENT and head and neck surgery.**

> **Assistant Professor at the FMOS**

> **ENT trainer at the INFSS**

> **Hospital practitioner at the Gabriel Toure University Hospital**

> **Member of the Malian ENT Society**

> **Member of the Beninese-Togolese ENT Society**

Dear Master,

It was with simplicity and humility that you responded favourably to our request to sit on this jury. By appreciating our modest work, you have effectively contributed to its indispensable improvement.

We are grateful for your presence here today and for all your help to us.

TO OUR MASTER AND CO-DIRECTOR DR. BROULAYE SAMAKE:

> **Specialist in anaesthesia and intensive care at the Gabriel Toure University Hospital;**

> **Assistant Master at the FMOS ;**

> **Head of the anaesthesia department at the Gabriel Toure University Hospital;**

> **Member of the Society of Anaesthesia, Resuscitation and Emergency Medicine of Mali (SARMU- MALI);**

> **Member of SARANF.**

Dear Master,

You have shown your confidence in us by entrusting us with this work. We have benefited from your scientific experience and your pertinent criticism. Your scientific rigour, your assiduity in your work, your availability and your sense of abnegation make you an exemplary teacher. Allow us to renew to you, dear master, in this happy circumstance, our gratitude and our best wishes for a long and enriching career.

TO OUR MASTER AND THESIS DIRECTOR
PROFESSOR DIENEBA DOUMBIA:
> **Lecturer in anaesthesia and intensive care ;**
> **Emergency and Disaster Physician ;**
> **Professor of Anaesthesia and Intensive Care at the FMOS;**
> **Head of the medical-surgical emergency department at the CHU du point-G;**
> **Member of SARMU-MALI;**
> **Member of SARANF.**
Dear Master,

We thank you for having accepted to ding this work. Your simplicity, your easy approach, your kindness, your rigour and your love for scientific work make you a respected and exemplary teacher.

Please accept our sincere thanks and deepest gratitude.

I. INTRODUCTION

Postoperative Nausea and Vomiting (PONV) is the term used to describe the nausea and vomiting that occurs in the first 24 hours after surgery [1]. From the patients' point of view, pain, nausea and vomiting are perceived as their most important concerns during the postoperative period [2]. In fact, vomiting is the most important postoperative complication for the patient, with pain and nausea coming second and third respectively [3]. The etiology of PONV is multifactorial. It is related to the type of surgery, duration of surgery, anaesthetic agents and techniques, postoperative analgesia and the physical and psychological state of the patient. The factors determining PONV are related to the patient's condition and medical and surgical history [8]. Following **PALAZZO** who identified three major risk factors [9], **APFEL** developed a universally accepted prediction score with four key risk factors: female gender, postoperative analgesia with opioids, postoperative emesis history and non-smoking [10]. Globally, **GAN** found that on average 30% of surgical patients experienced postoperative nausea and vomiting [6]. If 30% of surgery is performed on an outpatient basis and on average 1% of these patients require hospitalisation due to uncontrollable PONV, this results in 18,000 patients in France per year requiring unexpected hospitalisation due to these side effects [7]. In Mali, in a study carried out at the Gabriel Toure Hospital University Hospital, **TALA** found an average incidence of PONV in the order of 47.6% in ENT surgery **(cervicomaxillofacial)** [5].

PONV can develop into complications. These include inhalation of gastric contents or Mendelson's syndrome, suture loosening, Mallory-Weiss syndrome, alkalosis and hypokalemia, prolonged stay in the postoperative surveillance room, prolonged hospital stay [4]. In the **TALA Talon** study of 230 patients, 5.5% and 2.8% with PONV respectively had suture loosening and Mendelson syndrome [5].

Postoperative nausea and vomiting is not a life-threatening condition as it is rarely fatal and never becomes chronic. However, it is a real public health concern, especially since according to **VAN WIJK** patients tolerate pain better than PONV [11].

HILL proved the efficacy of Droperidol at a dosage of 0.625 mg to 1.25 mg in monotherapy [12].

Antiemetic prophylaxis appears to be more cost-effective than treatment of established symptoms in cases of high risk of PONV [13], especially in view of the limited resources available in African countries for the management of PONV, particularly in Mali. The objective of this study was to verify the value of dexamethasone for PONV prophylaxis in ENT surgery.

II. OBJECTIVES

<u>GENERAL OBJECTIVE</u> :

Study the interest of dexamethasone in the prevention of postoperative nausea and vomiting in ENT surgery at the Gabriel Toure University Hospital

<u>SPECIFIC OBJECTIVES</u> :

J To evaluate the effect of Dexamethasone on the prevention of postoperative nausea and vomiting.

J To describe the characteristics of PONV in ENT surgery.

S Identify prognostic factors with or without prevention.

III- GENERAL

A. DEFINITIONS OF NAUSEA AND VOMITING

a. Definition of nausea

Nausea is an unpleasant feeling of wanting to vomit, often accompanied by ANS symptoms such as heat, cold sweat, sialorrhea, tachycardia, and diarrhea [14]. It corresponds to a feeling of discomfort or unease in the stomach that results in choking or the urge to vomit.

It may be temporary and precede vomiting, or it may be permanent, which makes it a more painful symptom the longer it lasts.

b. Definition of vomiting

Vomiting or emesis is defined as an act of active discharge of gastrointestinal contents through the mouth. It results from a painful effort combining contractions not only of the abdominal muscles and the diaphragm but also digestive spasms with opening of the cardia [14]. It is accompanied by reflex changes in breathing and manifestations of vagal hyperarousal with hyper salivation and bradycardia.

c. Postoperative Nausea and Vomiting (PONV):

PONV refers to nausea and vomiting occurring within the first 24 hours after surgery [1].

B. Pathophysiology of nausea and vomiting.

Two brain regions are involved in the control of nausea and vomiting:

-A central, main area within the hematoencephalic barrier: the vomiting centre

-A zone outside the hemato-encephalic barrier: the chemoreceptive trigger zone (CTZ)

a. Vomiting centre (Figure 1a).

The vomiting centre corresponds to the area located in the lateral reticular formation of the spinal cord (elongated part of the mesencephalon or solitary nucleus region) and comprises a series of motor nuclei, including the nucleus ambiguus, the ventral and dorsal respiratory nucleus groups, and the dorsal motor nucleus of the vagus nerve. This area is responsible for the control and coordination of vomiting [15].

The respiratory response is characterised by simultaneous contraction of the diaphragm, abdominal muscles and expiratory intercostal muscles.

The digestive response results from the giant retrograde contraction of the small intestine and gastric antrum, the relaxation of the gastric fundus and thoracic resophagus, and the retrograde contraction of the cervical resophagus. Research suggests that the sensation of nausea is related to the inferior frontal gyrus of the cerebral cortex.

The neurochemistry of the vomiting centre is complex, involving over 30 neurotransmitters. Two of these, acetylcholine and histamine, are particularly important because drugs that antagonise these substances have a central effect on PONV. Most of the neuroreceptors involved are excitatory, i.e. they produce nausea and vomiting when stimulated, e.g. the receptors for histamine type 1, serotonin type 2 and muscarinic cholinergics. However, there are inhibitory neuroreceptors (ц opioid receptors). The Vomiting Centre is solicited by direct and indirect afferent pathways:

a.1 Direct afferents: come from different levels [16]:

> Peripheral level :

• The otorhino pharynx which carries tactile, olfactory and gustatory sensations and explains the vomiting caused by bad smells or foods that arouse disgust.

• The bronchial tree which accounts for vomiting caused by bronchial congestion or coughing fits.

• The digestive tract with the intervention of mechanoreceptors and chemoreceptors.

> Central level :

• The cerebral cortex which explains the important part played by the higher functions.

• The vestibular nuclei, which are very much involved in motion sickness and vertigo.

• The meninges.

a.2 Indirect afferents: by stimulation of the trigger zone located in the area postrema (central level).

The efferent pathways of vomiting are the *phrenic nerves* to the diaphragm, the *spinal nerves* to the abdominal musculature, and the *visceral nerves* efferent to the stomach and resophagus.

The neuroreceptors involved in the Vomiting Centre are of two types: *excitatory receptors* (type 1 histamine, muscarinic cholinergic and type 2 serotoninergic receptors) and *inhibitory receptors* (ц opioid receptors).

Distension of the walls of the gastrointestinal tract results in stimulation of the Vomiting Centre via the vagus nerve (X nerve), which triggers the vomiting reflex [17].

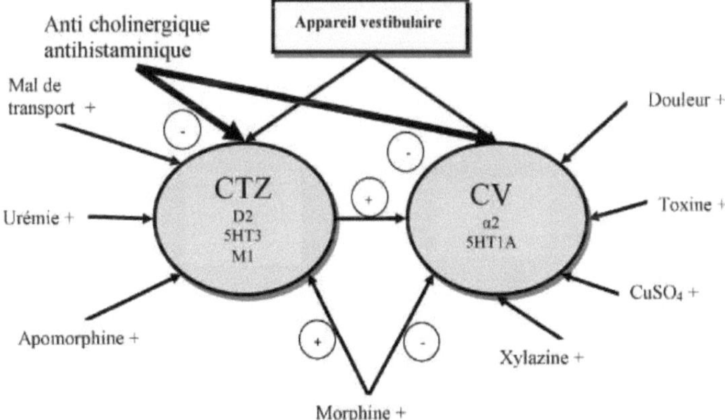

Figure 1a. *The vomiting centre* (VC) and *chemoreceptor zones* (CTZ) are stimulated or inhibited by many nerve factors and chemicals.

b. Chemoreceptor Zone (CTZ) (Figure 1b)

The chemoreceptor zone, also known as the *Chemoceptive Trigger* Zone (CTZ), is located in the area postrema, on the floor of the fourth ventricle and outside the hemato-encephalic barrier. The afferents to the Vomiting Centre pass through this area, but not exclusively. However, destruction of this Chemoreceptor Zone abolishes the emetic response to intravenously applied apomorphine or to certain cardiac glycosides [18].

Type 2 dopamine receptors (D2) are stimulated by high plasma concentrations of emetic substances such as calcium ions, urea, morphine, and digoxin. It also has an excitatory influence on the vestibule and vagus nerve: the neuroreceptors involved are D2 and the serotonin type 3 (5-HT3) receptor (excitatory).

The trigger zone can also be stimulated by irradiation, opiates and bacterial toxins.

Activation of the chemoreceptor area causes efferent impulses to travel to the vomiting centre, which in turn triggers vomiting.

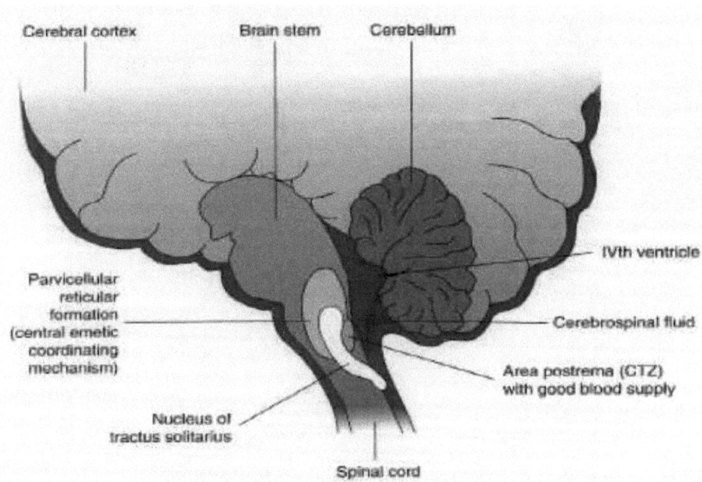

Figure 1b: *Chemoreceptor zone in the area postrema [18]*

c. **Vestibular and labyrinthine apparatus**

This device, located in the inner ear, has an excitatory influence on the vomiting centre and the trigger zone. It is activated by movements and changes in the environment.

The neuroreceptors involved at this level are *histamine type 1 (h1)*, *muscarinic cholinergic* (Achm) and *serotonin type 1A* (5-HT1A) *receptors*.

d. <u>Cerebral cortex and limbic system</u>

The limbic system is made up of the limbic and intralimbic convolutions and the olfactory lobe and plays a role in emotions.

The neurotransmitters involved are *histamine, q-acid* and *aminobutyric acid* (GABA) and *acetylcholine*.

Vomiting occurs as a result of electrical stimulation of the amygdala, olfactory tubercle, septum, fornix, anterior ventral thalamic nucleus, and the supraoptic region of the hypothalamus [19].

e. Visceral organs (Figure 2)

e.1 Creur

Through the vagus nerve, the voltage receptors (baroreceptors) located in the left ventricle are probably the ones that are stimulated, giving rise to excitatory nerve impulses. This could explain the nausea and vomiting associated with myocardial ischemia and vasovagal syncope [19].

e.2 Lungs

In the lungs, there are receptors whose stimulation via the vagus nerve gives rise to a tonic inhibitory impulse of gagging and vomiting [19].

e.3 Digestive tract

In the stomach and the proximal small intestine, an influx is produced by the afferent route via the vagus nerve. But for the small intestine in general, the impulse is generated by this route via the splanchnic nerves and the spinal cord. This is due to the presence of *mechanoreceptors in* the stomach, jejunum and ileum, whose stimulation by brushing, distension, compression and obstruction can cause nausea and vomiting.

The presence of *chemoreceptors* in the stomach, jejunum and ileum (which may exist in the mucosa as well as in the serosa), explains the nausea associated with peritonitis.

Their stimulation probably leads to the release of serotonin from the enterochromaffin cells, and activates the 5-HT4 receptors. The neuroreceptors are Dopaminergic type 2 (D2), Serotoninergic type 3 (5-HT3) and type 4 (5-HT4): which is the exciter.

Stress, anxiety and nausea from any cause induce a delay in gastric emptying via dopaminergic receptors located on interneurons in the myenteric plexus.

5-HT3 receptors are involved in emesis secondary to chemotherapy and radiotherapy, but not in emesis secondary to abdominal distension [19].

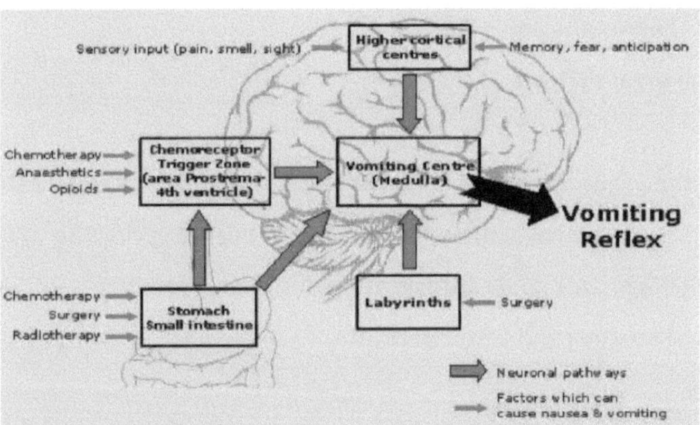

Figure 2: **Factors influencing vomiting.** *The Vomiting Centre can be directly stimulated by a variety of information from the digestive tract (stomach) or other organs such as the inner ear. The Vomiting Centre can also be stimulated inter-centrally by the "Chemosensitive Zone", which in turn can be stimulated by various clinical stimuli, including certain drugs.*

f. Mechanism of nausea and vomiting (Figure 3)

Nausea is usually associated with decreased motor activity in the stomach, duodenum and small intestine. The sensation of nausea is thought to be related to the inferior frontal gyrus of the cerebral cortex.

After a phase of nausea and a brief interval of retching, a sequence of involuntary visceral movements causes the vomiting itself. The phenomenon of forced ejection depends primarily on the abdominal musculature. Coinciding with a relaxation of the gastric fundus and gastroresophageal sphincter, a sudden increase in abdominal pressure is caused by a forced contraction of the descending diaphragm. Ventilation stops and the gastric and resophageal sphincters relax. Increased intra-thoracic pressure pushes the resophageal contents into the mouth. A reversal of the normal direction of resophageal peristalsis plays a role in this process: a reflex of elevation of the soft palate during vomiting prevents entry of the expelled material into the nasopharynx, while a reflex of closure of the glottis and inhibition of breathing prevents expulsion to the lungs. Thus, this mechanism sends the food bolus upwards into the stomach with increased salivation [20] <u>Clinical contexts of nausea and vomiting</u>

a. **<u>Postoperative nausea and vomiting</u>**

PONV, as the name suggests, occurs after surgery. It is considered a postoperative complication. Many factors are involved in the onset of postoperative nausea and vomiting. These include fluctuations in blood pressure and volume as well as the patient's position and certain movements [21]. It is recognised that the physical actions and manipulations of abdominal surgery lead to an effusion of various humoral substances that would trigger the nausea reflex via stimulation of 5-HT3 receptors in the vagus nerve domain.

b. **<u>Vomiting and intracranial hypertension</u>**

According to the **Monro-Kellie** hypothesis, intracranial pressure increases when one of the three components of the cranial cavity (blood, brain tissue, cerebrospinal fluid) increases in volume without a compensatory decrease in another component. Various clinical conditions are associated with increased intracranial pressure. These include tumours, cranial vault lesions, secondary lesions (cerebral oedema and haemorrhages), infections (e.g. meningitis and encephalitis) or cerebral pseudotumour. Vomiting, with or without nausea, may accompany these conditions once a critical value of intracranial volume is exceeded. **Epidemiology of postoperative nausea and vomiting**

a. **Impacts**

Nausea and vomiting are particularly painful, dreaded and common side effects of surgery.

Although rarely fatal and never becoming chronic, postoperative nausea and vomiting can be a significant stressor and discomfort for the patient.

Approximately 30% of all patients experience postoperative nausea and vomiting (PONV), and in some risk groups this incidence may be as high as 80% [22].

The frequency of postoperative nausea and vomiting varies between studies, with an average of around 25-30% [23].

In a study published by the Faculty of Medicine U.L.P. of Strasbourg, PONV occurs in 10% of patients admitted to the ICU [24]. According to KOIVURANTA, the incidence of PONV in the ICU is 20%, including 5% for vomiting alone [25]. BASTIA et al. found, in a study of 266 patients, that 33 of them, or 12.4% of the patients, had experienced PONV in the operating theatre [26].

In reality, results may differ in different settings. For example, the separate study of the incidence of nausea and vomiting resulted in a 50% incidence rate of PONV after halogen anaesthesia, half of which was vomiting [27]. It is one of the main causes of unplanned readmission after ambulatory surgery [28]. The readmission rate of patients with treatment-refractory PONV is estimated to be between 0.2 and 2% [7]. In ophthalmic surgery, the incidence of PONV remains very high: TRAMER found a rate of 50-60% [29] and van den BERG an incidence of 37-85% [30].

b. <u>Land and risk factors</u>

b.1 Factors related to the surgery

The incidence of PONV after general anaesthesia is directly influenced by the surgical site and certain surgical procedures.

b.2 Type of high-risk surgery

Laparoscopic abdominal surgery, particularly of the gynaecological sphere, is associated with a high incidence of PONV [31].

Stimulation of abdominal afferents by distension of the digestive tract elements and peritoneal traction probably plays a dominant role in the occurrence of PONV. The role of the menstrual cycle phase remains to be confirmed [32].

Ophthalmic surgery, particularly extraocular (strabismus) in children, is also a procedure associated with a high incidence of PONV. However, it appears that surgical technique is the main determinant [33].

ENT, face and neck surgery is also a high risk procedure. Direct stimulation of vestibular and/or vagal afferents in particular seems to explain the high incidence of PONV.

b.3 Duration of the surgery

The incidence of PONV increases with the duration of the surgical procedure [34]. The progressive increase in the response to surgical stress (adrenergic effect), as well as the accumulation of potentially emetogenic anaesthetic agents (e.g. halogen vapours or morphine), may favour the development of these adverse effects.

b.4 Anesthesia-related factors

> The premedication

- **Opiates**: There is clear evidence that the use of morphine as a premedication increases the risk of PONV [35]. Today, the trend in anaesthesiology is to no longer routinely give opiates as premedication.

- **Anticholinergics**: The systematic use of atropine or glycopyrrolate as a premedication has not been the case for some years; due to their unpleasant side effects and long duration, their use is limited to a few specific situations such as strabismus surgery. The antiemetic action of anticholinergics is central; indeed, in a double-blind study comparing atropine or glycopyrrolate, it was found that the latter was associated with twice the incidence of PONV [36].

- **Benzodiazepines**: This class of drugs is the most commonly used in premedication. At present, there are no studies suggesting the intrinsic antiemetic properties of benzodiazepines. However, it is well established that their anxiolytic action may be useful in attenuating the release of stress hormones associated with preoperative anxiety and indirectly play a favourable preventive role on PONV.

> The anaesthetic technique

Spinal anaesthesia: The incidence of PONV after spinal anaesthesia is generally lower than after general anaesthesia, due to the absence of agents

Int^ret of dexamëthasone in the prevention of PONV in ENT surgery volatile and opiates. However, this low incidence is a reality if complications such as hypotension or high block are avoided [37]. CARPENTER studied the incidence of PONV after spinal surgery prospectively in nearly 1000 patients. Nausea was noted in 18% and vomiting in 7% of the group [38]. Risk factors associated with PONV were: block above the T5 vertebra, a heart rate of 60 beats - min^{-1} prior to local anaesthetic infiltration, hypotension and the use of procaine as a local anaesthetic.

Peri-medullary anaesthesia: This significantly reduces the risk of PONV compared with either halogen or intravenous anaesthesia [39]. This technique is associated with the lowest incidence of PONV, statistically lower than that observed after general anaesthesia or spinal anaesthesia and represents the best anaesthetic technique for PONV prevention [40].

Total intravenous anaesthesia (*TIVA*): plays a role in reducing the incidence of PONV. Many studies corroborate this hypothesis. RAFTERY [41] studied patients after assisted conception. He clearly demonstrated that these women who received TIVA had significantly less PONV than those who received enflurane for maintenance: 7 versus 51% after 30 min and 34 versus 67% at 6^e hours postoperatively. GUNAWARDENE [42] studied the incidence of PONV in patients after minor gynecological surgery who received either TIVA, propofol/air or propofol/enflurane/N2O. The enflurane group showed the highest incidence of PONV (10%) while the propofol/air (TIVA) and propofol/N2O groups were lower (0% and 4% respectively).

> **Hypnotics.**

The incidence of PONV is greatly increased with ketamine. Similarly, PONV is three times more frequent with etomidate than with thiopental or methohexital [40]. KORTILLA has shown that the incidence of PONV is significantly reduced in ambulatory surgical patients who received propofol as an inducer compared to thiopental [43].

> **Gases or halogens.**

- **Role of nitrous oxide (N2O):** N2O promotes PONV either by decreasing middle ear pressure on awakening or by stimulating vestibular afferences by traction on the round window membrane [44]. In laparoscopic ambulatory surgery, PONV is significantly reduced if nitrous oxide is not included in the anaesthetic protocol. MELNICK and JOHNSON confirm this hypothesis by showing that the addition of N2O to the oxygen/isoflurane mixture increases the incidence of PONV [45]. APFEL identifies nitrous oxide and halogen vapours in general as the main risk factor for postoperative vomiting [46]. In contrast to recent studies in patients after laparoscopic gynaecological surgery, however, HORVOKA did not find a detrimental effect of N2O on PONV [47].

The omission of N2O from the anaesthetic protocol is still advisable.

> **Gastric emptying before extubation**

Insertion of a nasogastric tube to empty the stomach gives conflicting results on the incidence of PONV. The concept of gastric decompression stems from the experience that PONV was more common in women manually ventilated by inexperienced anaesthetists [48].

The benefit of gastric decompression on PONV had been shown by JANHUNEN and TAMMISTO [49] in patients after cholecystectomy. However, HOVARKA [50] did not note the benefits of this practice in 201 patients after laparotomy hysterectomy and the results of a meta-analysis no longer justify its systematic use in abdominopelvic surgery [51].

Routine insertion of a gastric tube is not an effective method of PONV; rather, nasopharyngeal stimulation of the tube itself or its presence in the duodenum is a potent stimulus for the onset of PONV. Similarly, to minimise pharyngeal stimulation, it is recommended that the nasogastric tube be placed after induction of anaesthesia and removed before extubation.

> **Decuritization**

The administration of atropine and neostigmine is associated with an increase in PONV despite the antiemetic action of atropine, suggesting an emetic effect of neostigmine [52].

> **Post-operative analgesia**

The interdependence between immediate postoperative pain and the incidence of PONV has been suggested by ANDERSEN and KROGH [53], a relationship found by JAKOBSSON [54]. PARNASS [55] studied the incidence of PONV and postoperative pain in patients after arthroscopy: no significant difference between PONV and the presence or absence of pain was observed.

Several authors have noted that PONV is rarely directly related to the intensity of postoperative pain. Administered opiates are more of a trigger than a preventative factor for PONV.

> Other peroperative factors

The use of 20 ml/kg of **crystalloid** during anaesthesia in ambulatory surgery would decrease the incidence of PONV and vertigo [56].

Mask ventilation would not be a contributing cause of PONV [57].

Early mobilisation and **oral rehydration** of patients would favour the occurrence of PONV [56]. This last measure is no longer part of the compulsory criteria for surgical discharge [58].

b.5 Patient-related factors

> Age

The incidence of PONV is higher in the paediatric population with a peak in pre-adolescence [40]. In contrast, ageing would decrease the risk of PONV [28, 59], although this factor has not been found in other studies [60, 26]. Nevertheless, BADAOUI, in a study of 145 patients aged 18 years and over, found that 69.4% of the subjects who presented with vomiting were under 60 years of age, with the oldest constituting only 30.5% of cases [61].

> Gender

The risk of PONV is higher in women during the active genital period between the ages of 11 and 55 [62, 26, 28, 34, 46, 59].

Variations in female hormone levels have been implicated as a causal factor. However, the relationship between cycle time and PONV is still very controversial.

HONKAVAARA found that the incidence of PONV was higher in the luteal phase [63], while BEATTIE found a correlation between PONV and menstruation up to day 8^{e} [64]. No hormonal assays have been performed to corroborate these results. However, **RAMSAY**, in patients taking oral contraceptives, found a peak of PONV between 9eme and 15eme days [65]. He suggests instead the involvement of restrogens.

> Weight

Weight overload is classically implicated as a factor in PONV [24]. The difficulty in ventilating these patients with a mask, the role of the fat mass as a reservoir for anaesthetic agents and gastrointestinal disorders are the usual explanations. Also, eostrogen hypersecretion by adipocytes is incriminated [66].

However, some studies do not consider increased body mass index as a risk factor for PONV [34, 67].

> **Transport diseases and PONV antecedents**

This group represents patients with a low threshold for PONV. It is suggested that these patients have developed a hyperstimulated reflex arc and/or have increased vestibular sensitivity in the middle ear.

All analyses show that motion sickness or a history of PONV doubles the risk of PONV [62, 60, 26, 28, 46, 59].

> **Anxiety**

The increased incidence of PONV in patients with high levels of anxiety is a well-known phenomenon among anaesthesiologists [40]. Anxiety is associated with increased stress hormones and there is a causal relationship with adrenergic stimulation.

However, some authors do not consider anxiety to be a relevant contributing factor in adults [62].

> **Power supply**

Prolonged preoperative fasting, or recent feeding, may increase the incidence of PONV [66].

> **Associated diseases**

Any damage associated with a motility disorder of the gastrointestinal tract may favour the occurrence of PONV [40]. In the context of a diabetic patient, the subject may present with pylorospasm, antral hypomotility and intrinsic neuropathy.

> **Special status**

Being a non-smoker significantly increases the incidence of PONV [60, 67]. The biological basis of the protective effect of smoking remains unknown, but it is likely that nicotine has anti-emetic properties and that its habituation decreases the probability of PONV [67]. However, the influence of nicotine seems to be less than that of female gender (odds ratio 2) [60, 26, 34, 46].

E.   PONV prediction scores

a.   Prediction scores

There are currently 5 PONV prediction scores:

PALAZZO was the first to apply the logistic regression technique [62] in orthopaedic surgery patients. A validation of this score on 400 patients suggested that this model could be transferred to other types of surgery [68].

The Sinclair score [59], constructed from an outpatient surgical population, is unique in that it includes patient, surgical and anaesthetic risk factors.

The Junger score [69] quantifies risk factors for predicting the need for PONV treatment based on retrospective analysis.

The Koivuranta score [26] confirms the importance of patient-related risk factors and calculates a discriminatory power. In addition, this score shows that simplification by reducing the number of risk factors to 5 would not alter the quality of their score, while allowing for more practical daily use.

The Apfel score [60] was designed to investigate whether risk scores from one centre could be valid in another centre and whether they could be simplified without losing discriminatory power. This score resulted in the retention of only 4 risk factors: female gender, history of motion sickness or PONV, non-smoker and receiving morphine postoperatively.

b.   Comparison of prediction scores

The PALAZZO and SINCLAIR scores underestimate the incidence of PONV by about 30% [28]. The PALAZZO score shows a lower discriminatory power than the other scores [70].

Only the APFEL and KOIVURANTA scores have satisfactory discriminatory power and calibration [28, 71].

The simplified APFEL score, due to its performance, ease of use and reproducibility, represents a very useful tool in daily practice and in clinical research [27, 70].

Table l.Simplified prediction scores for postoperative nausea and vomiting [72].

Risk factor	Score of Apfel et al	Score of Koivuranta et al
Female sex	+	+
History of PONV	}+	+
Travel sickness		+
Non-smoker	+	+
Post-operative morphine	+	-
Anaesthesia time > 60min	%	+
Discriminant power (AUC ROC)	0,68-0,71	0,70-0,71
Number of factors	PONV risk in (%) by number of factors	
0	<10	17
1	21	18
2	39	42
3	61	54
4	79	74
5	%	87

The Apfel and Koivuranta scores are calculated by assessing for a given patient the number of criteria that are met. The Apfel score comprises 4 criteria and the Koivuranta score 5. They have comparable discriminatory power and allow a quantified estimate of the risk of PONV.

c.   **The contribution of prediction scores**

This means that the probability of correctly predicting, on an individual basis, which patients will suffer from PONV and which will not is 80% maximum.

Adding predictive factors up to 7 to the simplified scores would not improve their discriminatory power, except if a significant risk factor (i.e. with a probability ratio >4) were found.

F.   **Complications of PONV**

Although the occurrence of PONV complications is rare [24], their severity is always formidable, hence the importance of being aware of them.

The most common complications include [40, 16]:

a. **Bronchial inhalation (Mendelson's syndrome):** an acute respiratory syndrome characterised by the irruption of gastric fluid into the tracheobronchial tree, most often in the perioperative period. It is characterised by a so-called "deglutition" pneumopathy, usually of the right base, and/or an acute pulmonary lesion-like redness.

b. **Suture loosening**

c. **Intraocular and skin bleeding** (during plastic surgery)

d. **Mallory-Weiss syndrome (cardiac ulceration)** is characterised by dilatation of the mucosa of the lower resophagus and cardia. It is responsible for digestive bleeding.

e. **Oesophageal and hypogastric burns**: these are caused by exposure to hydrochloric acid during vomiting.

f. **Traumatic rupture of the resophagus (Boerhaave syndrome)**.

g. **Metabolic alkalosis**: repeated vomiting leads to a loss of acids from the digestive tract, resulting in an increase in plasma bicarbonate concentration. Metabolic alkalosis is manifested by myoclonic jerks, and the presence of Chvostek's sign (patent muscle contraction of the superior bundle of the orbicularis of the lips and the buccinator).

h. **Hypokalemia (potassium level<3mmol/l)**: is caused by vomiting and aggravated by metabolic alkalosis.

i. **Other metabolic disorders**: dehydration, malnutrition, hypocalcemia, risk of renal failure.

j. **Prolongation of the recovery room stay** in case of early PONV with an Aldrete recovery score < 7/10.

k. The impact on **mood** and **appetite**: a patient who does not eat is a patient who is unwell.

G. Treatment of PONV

a. Therapeutic means

a.1 Pharmacological treatment

Drugs recognised as antiemetic agents and used in the management of PONV are generally grouped according to the type of receptor on which they act *(see Table I)*.

Table I: *Antiemetics: dosage and route of administration*

Drugs	Group	Dose, route, frequency of administration
Dexamëthasone	corticosteroi'de	6-10mg IV as preferred combination
Ondansëtron	5-HT3 antagonist	4-8mg PO IM or IV, 24mg max per 24 hours 16mg PO, 1 hour pre-op in one dose
Granisëtron	5-HT3 antagonist	1mg IV, 2mg max per 24 hours
Dompëridone	D2 antagonist	10 -20 mg PO, 60 mg max per 24 hours 60 mg IR every 4 to 8 hours
Dropëridol	D2 antagonist	0.5-1.25mg IV every 8 hours 2.5-5mg PO every 8 hours
Mëtoclopramide	D2 antagonist	10 mg IM or IV every 6 hours
prochlorperazine	D2 antagonist	12.5 mg PO or IM every 6 hours 25 mg IR as initial dose 3 mg oral preparation available
Atropine	Anticholinergic	0.3-0.6 mg IM or IV, 30-60 min pre op
Hyoscine	Anticholinergic	0.2-0.4 mg SC or IM every 6 hours 1 mg transdermal patch, duration 72h
Promethazine	Antihistamine	25 mg PO, 100 mg max per 24h
cyclizine	Antihistamine	50 mg PO IM, IV every 8 hours

.D2= dopaminergic type 2; 5-HT3: serotoninergic type 3; IM= intramuscular; IV= intravenous; SC= subcutaneous; PO= per os.

A meta-analysis of 54 double-blind, randomised, controlled studies was able to prove the previously assumed superiority of ondansetron and droperidol over metoclopramide [71].

Ondansetron has more antiemetic than anti-nausea properties, whereas droperidol has more anti-nausea than anti-nausea properties. However, ondansetron does not have a good effect against morphine-induced PONV.

Prevention should be reserved for high risk patients *(see Figure 5)*. Prophylactic administration of a cocktail before extubation is more effective than administration at induction [73].

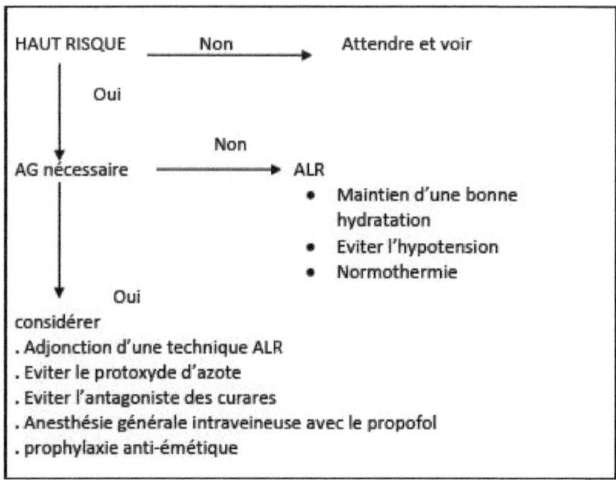

Maintaining good hydration
Avoiding hypotension
Normothermie
"Yes consider . Addition of ALR technique . Avoid nitrous oxide . Avoid curare antagonist . Intravenous general anaesthesia with propofol .

Figure 5: Prevention of PONV.

GA= General Anaesthesia; LRA= Local Anaesthesia.

H. **Corticoids and PONV**

a. **Definition and classification**

Corticoids are natural steroid hormones, derived from cholesterol, whose production is stimulated by ACTH released in a nocturnal cycle by the anterior lobe of the pituitary gland, secreted in humans by the cortex of the suprarenal gland. This superficial part of the gland produces :

-Glucocorticoids (cortisol) which have anti-inflammatory properties and an action on protein and carbohydrate metabolism.

-Mineralocorticoids (mainly aldosterone) which act on water and salt regulation in the body

-Androgens.

In general, when we speak of "corticoids", we are referring to glucocorticoids, whether natural or synthetic.

Glucocorticoids have a higher activity to allow a better anti-inflammatory action and their mineralocorticoid effects are very reduced. They are used in other therapeutic indications and are defined as:

- Short-acting corticoids (prednisone, prednisolone, methylprednisolone): anti-inflammatory potency of 4-5 (measured by reference to cortisol of 1)

- Intermediate-effect corticoids (triamcinolone, paramethasone): with an inflammatory power of 5 to 10

- Long-acting corticoids (betamethasone, dexamethasone, cortivazol) with an inflammatory power of 25-30 (up to 60 for cortivazol). [79]

Corticosteroids, and in particular dexamethasone, reduce the incidence of postoperative nausea and vomiting, a fact that is now well established both by meta-analyses of all studies devoted to this effect and all surgical procedures and also specifically during a particular procedure such as tonsillectomy [74].

b. Mechanism of action

The mechanism of dexamethasone's antiemetic action is not clearly established. The hypothesis is that it acts centrally by inhibiting either prostaglandin synthesis or endorphin release [75]. Glucocorticoids may also decrease cerebral serotonin levels or prevent its release from the digestive tract.

c. Efficiency

c.1 Corticosteroids for PONV prophylaxis

The superiority of dexamethasone over placebo in the prevention of PONV is clearly demonstrated. The efficacy of dexamethasone is broadly similar to that of 5HT3 receptor antagonists and droperidol in terms of both nausea and vomiting. Dexamethasone is more effective than metoclopramide in preventing PONV[76].

The relative risk of PONV is reduced by 80% after tonsillectomy [74]. The absolute rate of reduction after different types of surgery is about 25%, comparable to that of droperidol and setrons. [40]

c.2 Corticosteroids in combination with other antiemetics for PONV prophylaxis

The combination of dexamethasone with an AR-5HT3, droperidol or high dose metoclopramide is more effective than dexamethasone alone.

Recommendation: Dexamethasone is recommended for the prevention of PONV in patients at risk. In high-risk patients, combination with an AR-5HT3 and/or droperidol is recommended. [76]

c.3 Corticosteroids in PONV treatment

In the absence of literature, dexamethasone is not recommended for the treatment of PONV. However, this steroid may, in combination, reduce the incidence of recurrence of PONV episodes. [76]

d. Benefits of corticosteroids

Single-dose dexamethasone for the prevention of PONV is a simple, effective, well-tolerated and inexpensive solution. [76]

e. Disadvantages of corticosteroids

The increase in blood glucose after administration of dexamethasone has been found in diabetic and non-diabetic patients. Although the risk of infection has not been specifically evaluated, epidemiological data are reassuring in this indication. [76]

f. Corticosteroid administration protocols

f.1 Dose

Efficacy increases with dosage. The minimum effective dose of dexamethasone appears to be about 4 mg.

The recommended intravenous dose of dexamethasone for the management of PONV is between 4 and 8 mg. [76]

In paediatrics, dosages found in the literature vary by a factor of 10 (from 0.15 to 1.5 mg .kg), but a recent study showed that low doses (0.0625 mg .kg) are as effective in reducing the incidence of OPV as higher doses [77]. No side effects were found at the usual doses.

f.2 Time of administration

Because of its delayed onset of action, it is recommended that it be administered at the time of anaesthetic induction, which is more effective than administration at the end of the procedure [78].

IV METHODOLOGY

1. **Study framework :**

Our study took place in the ENT Surgery Department and the Department of Anaesthesia-Reanimation and Emergency Medicine of the Gabriel Toure University Hospital Centre (CHU) in Bamako.

The Gabriel Toure Hospital is one of the 3 national hospitals of the Republic of Mali. It is a former dispensary located in the commune III of the district of Bamako. It was established as a hospital on 17 February 1959 and owes its name to a student of the same name who died of the plague contracted from one of his patients. The CHU Gabriel Toure is located in the administrative centre of the city of Bamako in Commune III. It is bordered to the east by the Medina Coura district, to the west by the Ecole Nationale d'Ingenieur (ENI), to the north by the Armed Forces Headquarters and to the south by the railway station.

1.1 The Department of Anaesthesia, Resuscitation and Emergency Medicine

It is located in the south and has three parts: an anaesthesia part which covers all the anaesthetic activities of the hospital, an emergency part and an adult resuscitation part.

1.2 The ENT department

The ENT department is a medical-surgical department with two professors assisted by five ENT specialists from the university hospital.

In addition, the department has at its disposal for its daily functioning: 4 hospital interns and 8 doctors enrolled in DES; 6 medical assistants specialists in dexaméthasone in the prevention of PONV in ENT surgery, 2 health technicians, 1 management secretary, 1 surface technician, and students from the Faculty of Medicine and Odontostomatology (FMOS) of Bamako.

2. **Type and period of study :**

This was a randomised, single-blind study, involving hospital recruitment of patients who had undergone ENT surgery and were hospitalised in the ENT department of the CHU Gabriel TOURE.

This study took place over a period from November 2013 to May 2014

3. **Study population :**

The study included all patients admitted for ENT surgery

4. **Sampling :**

4.1 Inclusion criteria :

Any patient operated on for ENT pathology, scheduled in the operating theatre of the Gabriel Toure University Hospital and hospitalized for at least 24 hours in the postoperative period in this department.

4.2 Non-inclusion criteria :

> Any patient from a surgical department other than ENT,

> Any patient who is not hospitalized or who is hospitalized for less than 24 hours postoperatively.

> Any non-consenting patient.

> Any patient who has not been operated on in the ENT department of the Gabriel Toure University Hospital

> Patient with a contraindication to the use of dexamethasone.

> Patient who will present with nausea and vomiting beyond 24 hours.

4. 3. Sample size

The sample size was calculated using the formula :

$$N = (s^2 \, a \, X \, p \, Xq)/ \, p$$

N= minimum sample size.

s= Reduced deviation of the normal distribution, equal to 1.96 for a risk a=5%.

Confidence level = 95%.

P= relative frequency of a measurable event on the issue.

Q= complement of the probability p=1-q, q=1-p.

I= accuracy, varies between 2% and 8% (in medical studies).

P= 0.476 q=1-P q=1-0.476=0.524

N= (г'Л/.x Pxq)/P

Here: £=1.96 for a=5%.

P= 0,476

Q=0,524

I=8%
N= [(1.96)2x 0.476x0.524]/ (0.08)2 = 149 .716
N= 149.716 plus 5% margin of error

150 + 5%(150) = 150 + 8 = 158

N = 158

The required sample size was estimated at 158 cases.

5. Method

5.1 Selection method :

The draw was made in a random way

It was a method of drawing lots from a population, divided into two groups **A** and **B**:

- **Group A** contained all patients with an even enrolment number and this group will receive Dexamethasone as antiemetic prophylaxis at a dose of 4mg for patients under 80kg and 8mg for those over 80kg as a slow IV at induction.

- **Group B** contained all patients with an odd enrolment number and will not receive any anti-emetic prophylaxis.

5.2 Conduct of the study :

For each of the selected patients, the following parameters were studied:

> The general data, allowing :

- To provide information about the patient: identity (name and surname), age, sex, weight, place of residence, occupation.

> Clinical data, covering :

- Personal medical and surgical history of the patient, obstetrical history (for female patients),

- Lifestyle, diagnosis and indication for surgical treatment,
- identify preoperative feeding: type, schedule ;
- to collect post-intervention data on

PONV events: date and time of onset, place of onset, extent and aspects of nausea and vomiting.

> The procedure of the surgical act including :

- type and duration of surgery ;
- premedication administered ;
- anaesthetic products used ;

> clinical assessment demonstrating :

- postoperative analgesia performed ;
- the type of discomfort, its timing in the postoperative period and its impact on the patient's general condition;
- complications that may arise.

> The Apfel score: it classifies patients according to PONV risk factors. Thus we will identify the presence or absence of four major risk factors according to APFEL, namely female gender, history of PONV, non-smoking status and postoperative opioid use.

> The course of action and revolution is defined either by the possible therapeutic management of PONV, or by gastric emptying, or by therapeutic abstention and monitoring of the parameters.

All these steps will be accomplished with the cooperation of the staff of the ENT and Anaesthesia-Reanimation department of the Gabriel Toure Hospital.

6. Outcome: The outcome of our study was the occurrence of postoperative nausea and vomiting. PONV will be investigated through questioning of patients and/or their companions at the twenty-fourth hour after surgery by the investigator.

7. Treatment in case of PONV.

In our study, patients with more than 3 episodes of vomiting and those with postoperative nausea were treated with metopimazine (VOGALENE®), an antiemetic belonging to the chemical class of phenothiazines, which is characterised by its selective anti-dopaminergic activity (anti-apomorphine activity) due to its very limited passage through the hemato-encephalic barrier.

The dosage will be adapted according to the time and intensity of the disorder:

Adults: either 1 capsule (15mg) X 2 per day; or 1 suppository (5mg) X 3 per day; or 1 lyoc (7.5mg) X 2 to 4 per day; or lampoule (10mg) X 1 to 3 per day IM or slow IV, reducing the dose in elderly subjects or those with cardiovascular abnormalities

Children: 0.5 mg/kg/d in 2 to 3 doses, suppositories or oral suspension are recommended.

8. Data support.

All patients in our study were collated according to socio-demographic and clinical data, and then recorded on an individual survey form, which was tested and validated before the survey.

9. Data exploitation :

Data entry and analysis were performed with Microsoft Office Word 2007, Microsoft Office Excel 2007, SPSS 19.0 and Epi info 6.04. The statistical test used was Pearson's Chi-square^2 and Fisher's exact test. The significance level for our statistical tests was set at 0.05.

10. Ethical aspects

The study was carried out with the patient's consent and the confidentiality of the data was ensured by restricted access to the files.

V RESULTS

1. <u>Frequency :</u>

In our study, out of a total of 158 patients, **43** had postoperative nausea and/or vomiting, i.e. **27.22%**.

2. <u>Descriptive data:</u>

<u>Tableau I</u>   Distribution of patients by age group (N=158)

	Absolute frequencies	Relative frequencies
< 10 years	**39**	**24.7**
10-19 years	38	24.1
20-29 years	37	23.4
30-39 years old	26	16.5
40-49 years old	6	3.8
50-59 years	6	3.8
60-69 years	5	3.2
>70 years	1	.6
Total	158	100.0

24.7% of our patients were younger than 10 years. The mean age was 21.96 ± 15.40 years with extremes of 32 months and 72 years.

<u>Tableau II</u>   Distribution of patients by gender (N=158)

gender	Absolute frequencies	Relative frequencies
Male	55	34,8
Female	103	65,2
Total	158	100.0

The female sex was represented in 65.2% of cases

<u>Table III:</u> Distribution of patients by weight (n=158).

Weight (in kg)	Absolute frequencies	Relative frequencies(%)
< 10 Kg	4	2.5
10-19 kg	25	15.8
20-29 kg	14	8.9
30-39 kg	7	4.4
40-49 kg	11	7.0
50-59 kg	16	10.1
60-69 kg	**35**	**22.2**
70-79 kg	29	18.4
>80 kg	17	10.8
Total	158	100.0

22.2% of the patients had a weight between **60 and 69 kg**. The average weight was **50.58kg ± 24.31kg** with extremes of **6 and 94kg**.

Table IV: Distribution of patients by lifestyle (N=158).

Lifestyle	Absolute frequencies	Relative frequencies
Tobacco	8	5,1
Alcohol	1	0,6
The	26	16,5
No special features	123	77,8
Total	158	100

8 patients smoked tobacco.

Table V: Distribution of patients by origin (N=158)

Place of residence	Absolute frequencies	Relative frequencies
bamako	150	94,9
Interior	8	5,1
Total	158	100.0

94.9% of the patients lived in Bamako

Table VI: Distribution of patients according to ASA classification (N=158)

ASA	Workforce	Percentage
ASA 1	**146**	**92.4**
ASA 2	10	6.3
ASA 3	2	1.3
Total	158	100.0

92.4% of patients were **ASA 1**, i.e. 146

Table VII: Distribution of patients according to the number of risk factors

Apfel score	Workforce	Percentage
0	8	5.1
1	50	31.6
2	100	63.3
Total	158	100.0

100 patients or **63.3%** of our sample had **2** risk factors.

Table VIII: Distribution of patients according to the duration of the intervention

Duration of the intervention	Numbers	Percentage (%)
< 30 minutes	5132	.3
30-59 minutes	**5937**	**.3**
60-89 minutes 90-119	106.3	
minutes > 120 minutes	138.2	
	2515	.8
Total	158100	.0

37.3% of the interventions (**59**) lasted **less than 1 hour**. The average duration was **58.6 ± 39.66 min** with extremes of **20** and **190** min.

Table IX: Distribution of patients according to decurarisation (n=158).

decurarisation	Workforce	Percentage (%)
neostigmine	4	2.5
not done	**154**	**97.5**
Total	158	100.0

97.5% of our patients (**154**) did not undergo decurarisation.

Table X: Distribution of patients according to postoperative analgesia

Postoperative analgesia	Workforce	Percentage(%)
noramidopyrin	6	3.8
paracetamol	**147**	**93.0**
not done	3	1.9
acupan and paracetamol	2	1.3
Total	158	100.0

93% of patients (**147**) had received **paracetamol (perfalgan)**

Table XI: Distribution of patients according to the occurrence of PONV (n=158)

Type of discomfort	Numbers	Percentage(%)
nausea	1811 .4	
vomiting	127.6	
nausea and vomiting	138.2	
no	11572.8	
Total	158100	.0

27.2% of the patients had PONV (**43/158**).

Table XII: Distribution of patients by time of onset of PONV (n=43)

Time of appearance	Workforce	Percentage(%)
between 0 and 6 hours post operations	37	86.0
between 7 and 12 hours post-operatively	5	11.6
between 19 and 24 hours post-op	1	2.3
Total	43	100.0

86% of patients experienced PONV between 0 and 6 hours after surgery.

3. Analytical data

Table XIII: **Distribution of patients according to age group and antiemetic prophylaxis (N=158)**

BandGroup   AG Group B

age

	staff	Frequency(%)	staff	Frequency(%)
< 10 years	18	22,8	21	26.6
10-19 years	14	17,7	**24**	**30,4**
20-29 years	**20**	**25.3**	17	21,5
30-39 years old	15	19,0	11	13,9
40-49 years old	4	5,1	2	2,5
50-59 years	4	5,1	2	2.5
60-69 years	3	3,8	2	2,5
>70 years	1	1,3	0	0
Total	79	100	79	100

In group A, **25.3%** were aged between **20** and **29 years**.

The mean age was 25 **± 16.1 years** with extremes of **02 years** and **72 years**.

In group B, **30.4%** were aged between **10** and **19 years**.

The mean age was 19.3 **± 14.1 years** with extremes of **32 months** and **63 years**.

Table XIV: **Gender distribution of patients (n=158).**

gender	Group A	number of people	Group B	number of people	Total
Male	28	35.4	27	34.2	55(34,8%)
Female	51	64.6	52	65.8	103(**65,2%**)
Total	79	100	79	100	158(100%)

The female sex was represented in **65.2%** of cases. The sex ratio was 1.87 in favour of the female sex.

Table XV: **Distribution of patients by antiemetic** **weight and   prophylaxis**

(n=158)

Weight (in kg)	Group A		Group B	
	workforce	Frequency(%)	workforce	Frequency(%)
< 10	3	3,8	1	1,3
10-19	10	12,7	**15**	**19**
20-29	6	7,6	8	10,1
30-39	4	5,1	3	3,8

40-49	6	7,6	5	6,3
50-59	8	10,1	8	10,1
60-69	**20**	**25,3**	**15**	**19**
70-79	14	17,7	**15**	**19**
>80	8	10,1	9	11,4
Total	79	100	79	100

In group A, **25.3%** of the patients had a weight between **60 and 69 kg**.

In group B, **19%** of the patients weighed between **10 and 19 kg**, **60 and 69 kg** and **70 and 79 kg** each.

Table XVI: Distribution of patients by lifestyle (N=158).

Mode of life	Group A number of people		Group B number of people		Total
Tobacco	5	6,3	3	3,8	8(5,1%)
Alcohol	0	0	1	1,3	1(0,6%)
The	14	17,7	12	15,2	26(16,5%)
Without special	60	76 ,0	63	79,7	123(77,8%)
Total	79	100	79	100	158(100%)

8 patients smoked, i.e. **6.3%** of patients in group A and **3.8%** of those in group B.

Clinical data

Table XVII: Distribution of patients by medical history (N=158).

ATCDs
MEDICAL Group A Group B

	staff	Frequency(%)	staff	Frequency(%)
UGD	**7**	**8,9**	7	**8,9**
HTA	4	5,1	2	2,5
tuberculosis	1	1,3	0	0
asthma	2	2,5	0	0
other	1	1,3	6	7,6
without history	68	86,1	65	82,3

<u>Other medical history</u>: sickle cell disease(l); epilepsy(2); haemoglobinopathy(l); pneumonia(1); sinusitis(2)

7 patients in each group **(8.9%)** had a history of peptic ulcer disease

<u>**Table XVIII:**</u> **Distribution of patients according to ASA classification and antiemetic prophylaxis (N=158)**

patient classification according to ASA	Group A number of people	Frequency(%)	Group B effect if	Frequency(%)
ASA 1	**75**	**94.9**	**71**	**89,9**
ASA 2	3	3,8	7	8,8
ASA 3	1	1,3	1	1,3
Total	79	100	79	100

75 patients in group A (94.9%) were ASA 1 compared to 89.9% (71/79) in group B

<u>**Table XIX**</u>**: Distribution of patients according to the number of risk factors and anti-emetic prophylaxis.**

score of Apfel	Group	AG Group B	
	Actual Frequency(%)	Actual Frequency(%)	Total
0	45,	045 ,	18
1	2734 ,	22329,	150
2	4860 ,	85265,	8100
Total	7910079100158		

48 patients or **60.8%** had two risk factors in group A versus **65.8% (52/79)** in group B.

<u>**Table XX**</u>**: Distribution of patients according to pre-operative fasting.**

time between the last meal and the operation	AG Group BTotal Group		
	Actual Frequency(%)	Actual Frequency(%)	
less than 12	2126,	62227, 843(27,2%)	
hours between 12 and 6 p.m.	58 **73,4**	57 **72,**	**2115(72,8%)**
Total	7910079100158 (100%)		

72.8% of patients (**115**) had a pre-operative fasting time of ***between 12 and 18 hours***

Table XXI: Distribution of patients by operative diagnosis (N=158).

diagnosis per operative	Group A		Group B		Total
	staff	Frequency(%)	staff	Frequency(%)	
tonsillitis	43	54,4	50	63,3	93(58.9%)
otitis media chronicle	15	19	16	20,3	31(19,6%)
goitre	2	2,5	4	5,1	6(3,8%)
laryngeal tumour	3	3,8	0	0,0	3(1,9%)
purulent rhinorrhea	0	0,0	1	1,3	1(0,6%)
pharyngeal tumour	1	1,3	0	0,0	1(0,6%)
perforation tympanic	0	0,0	1	1,3	1(0,6%)
cleft lip	4	5,1	0	0,0	4(2,5%)
mass right laterocervical	1	1,3	0	0,0	1(0,6%)
rope polyp voice	0	0,0	1	1,3	1(0,6%)
mass anterocervical	1	1 ,3	0	0,0	1(0,6%)
adenoide vegetation	3	3,8	2	2,5	5(3,2%)
papillomatosis laryngee	0	0 ,0	1	1, 3	1(0,6%)
seromucosal otitis	3	3,8	0	0,0	3(1,9%)
laryngeal web	1	1,3	0	0,0	1(0,6%)
lingual mass	0	0,0	1	1,3	1(0,6%)
septal derivation	2	2,5	0	0,0	2(1,3%)
floor cyst oral	0	0,0	2	2,5	2(1,3%)
Total	79	100	79	100	158(100%)

58.6% of all patients underwent surgery for tonsillitis, **43** in group A **(54.4%)** and **50** in group B **(63.3%)**

Int^ret of dexamëthasone in the prevention of PONV in ENT surgery **19.6%** of the patients were operated for **chronic otitis media**, i.e. **31/158** (15/79 in group A and 16/79 in group B)

J **Perioperative period**

Table XXII: **Distribution of patients according to premedication (N=158).**

premedication	Group A		Group B headcount		
	staff	Frequency(%)		Frequency(%)	Total
Diazepam+Atropine	20	25,3	29	36,7	**49(31,0%)**
Atropine	8	10,1	8	10,1	**16(10,1%)**
Diazepam	19	24,1	11	13,9	**30(19,0%)**
No	32	40,5	31	39,2	63(39,9%)
Total	79	100	79	100	158(100%)

95 patients had received a premedication, i.e. **60.1%** of all patients. The combination of **diazepam and atropine** was used as premedication in 49 patients or **31.0%** of the sample.

All surgical procedures were performed under *general anaesthesia* (GA) during our study.

Table XXIII: **Distribution of patients according to anaesthetic products used**

Anesthetic products	Group A		Group B		Total
	staff	Frequency(%)	staff	Frequency (%)	
ketamine	35	44,3	24	30,4	59(37,3%)
propofol	31	39.2	31	39.2	62(39,2%)
thiopental	**30**	**38**	**37**	**46,8**	**67(42,4%)**
fentanyl	60	75,9	62	78,5	122(77,2%)
celocurine	28	35.4	32	40,5	60(38%)
vecuronium	29	36,7	31	39,2	60(38%)
halothane	44	55,7	36	45,6	**80(50,6%)**
isoflurane	14	17,7	26	32,9	**40(25,3%)**

120 patients received **anaesthetic gases** in maintenance, i.e. **75.95%**, of which

73.42% (58/79) were in group A and 78.48% (62/79) in group B.

Thiopental was the hypnotic used in anaesthetic induction with 42.4% or **38%** (30/79) in group A and **46.8%** (37/79) in group B.

122 patients had received **fentanyl**.

Table XXIV: Distribution of patients according to duration of surgery and antiemetic prophylaxis

| Duration of the intervention | Group A | | Group B | | |
	staff	Frequency(%)	staff	Frequency(%)	Total
< 30 minutes	28	35,4	23	29,1	51(32,3%)
30-59 minutes	24	30,4	35	44,3	**59(37,3%)**
60-89 minutes	7	8,9	3	3,8	10(6,3%)
90-119 minutes	6	7.6	7	8,9	13(8,2%)
> 120 minutes	14	17,7	11	13,9	25(15,8%)
Total	79	100	79	100	158(100%)

The intervention time of **30 to 59 minutes** was represented by **37.3%**, 30.4% in Group A and 44.3% in Group B.

Fisher's exact test p= 0.345

J Postoperative period

Table XXV: Distribution of patients according to time of return to food

| Post-operative dietary resumption | Group A Actual | | Group B | | |
		Frequency(%)	effect	if Frequence(%)	Total
0 to 6^e hours	**55**	69,6	**51**	64,6	**106(67,1%)**
7^e to 12th hour	**21**	26,6	**21**	26,6	**42(26,6%)**
13th to 18th hour	**0**	0	**5**	6,3	**5(3,2%)**
18th to 24th hour	3	3,8	2	2,5	5(3,2%)
Total	79	100	79	100	158(100%)

67.1% of the patients had resumed feeding at 6eme **hours**, i.e. **106** of whom **55** from group A and **51** from group B.

73

Table XXVI: Distribution of patients according to the occurrence of PONV with or without prophylaxis.

| Type of discomfort | Group A | | Group B | | |
	effective	Frequency(%)	effective	Frequency(%)	Total
nausea	6	7,6	12	15,2	18(11,4%)

	Group A f	%	Group B f	%	Total
vomiting	4	5,1	8	10,1	12(7,6%)
nausea and vomiting	5	6,3	8	10,1	13(8,2%)
NVPO	**15**	**19**	**28**	**35,4**	**43(17,2)**
no	64	81	51	64,6	115(72,8%)
Total	79	100	79	100	158(100%)

Fisher's exact test p= 0.031282018406852

Odds Ratio: 0.4292 95% confidence interval [0.1912; 0.9334].

18 patients had **nausea, i.e. 11.4%** of the sample, including **6** from group A **(7.6%)** and 12 from group B **(15.2%)**;

13 patients had **PONV, i.e. 8.2%** of the sample, including **5** patients in group A **(6.3%)** and **8** patients in group B **(10.1%)**

12 patients experienced **vomiting, i.e. 7.6%** of the sample, including **4** patients in group A **(5.1%)** and **8** patients in group B **(10.1%)**

Table XXVII: **Distribution of patients according to the nature of the vomiting (n=25)**

Aspect of vomiting	Group A effect f	Frequency(%)	Group B effectiveness f	Frequency(%)	Total
Liquid	3	33,3	2	12,5	5(20%)
Food	1	11,1	3	18,8	4(16%)
Hematic (reddish)	0	0	3	18,8	3(12%)
Bilious (green or yellowish)	5	**55,6**	**8**	50	**13(52%)**
Total	9	100	16	100	25(100%)

Chi-square^2 =3.182 p= 0.364 (Fisher's exact test P =0.529)

13 patients presented postoperative emesis with a **bilious appearance, i.e. 52%**, including **5** patients in group A and **8** patients in group B.

<u>**Table XXVIII:**</u> **Distribution of patients according to the number of episodes of vomiting.**

Number of vomits		Group A Actual Frequency(%)		Group B Actual Frequency(%)		Total
1 episode	**4**	44,4	**11**	68,8		**15(60%)**
2 episodes	**1**	11,1	**3**	18,8		**4(16%)**
3 episodes and more	**4**	44,4	**2**	12,5		**6(24%)**
Total	9	100	16	100		25(100%)

15 patients with OPV had only one episode of vomiting, i.e. **60%** of all OPV patients (15/25).

Of these 15 patients, **36.4%** had received dexamethasone, while **67.6%** had not.

Chi-square^2 =3.226ddl= 2 P= 0.199 (Fisher exact test P= 0.269)

<u>**Table XXIX:**</u> **Distribution of PONV according to anti-emetic treatment and prophylaxis**

Antiemetic treatment	*Group A N(%)*	*Group B N(%)*	*Total*
Yes	4 (36,4)	2(7,1)	6
No	**11 (63,6)**	**26 (92,9)**	**37**
Total	15	28	43

37 patients suffering from PONV did not require anti-emetic treatment, i.e. **86.0%, 63.6%** of whom were in group **A** compared with **92.9%** of those in group **B**. (Fisher's exact test P= 0.161; odd ratio = 4 .5391 I.C = (0.5574; 57.1145)

<u>**Table XXX:**</u> **Distribution of PONV according to food intake.**

Post-operative dietary resumption	nausea	vomiting	NVPO	No	Total
0 to 6^e hours	**14(77,8)**	9(75)	**4(30,8)**	79(68,7)	**106(67,1%)**
7^e a 12^e hour 13 to 18^e	**4(22,2)**	3(25)	**6(46,2)**	29(25,2)	**42(26,6%)**
hour	**0**	0	**3(23,1)**	2(1,7)	**5(3,2%)**
18ea 24th hour	0	0	0	5(4,3)	5(3,2%)

| Total | 18 | 12 | 13 | 115 | 158(100%) |

Fisher's exact test gives P=0.051350909902841

27 patients had **PONV before the** 6i^{eme} **hour** after resumption of feeding, i.e.

62.8% of those who had experienced discomfort

<u>Table XXXI</u>: PONV by diagnosis

intraoperative diagnosis	Type of discomfort				Total
	nausea	vomiting	Nausea and vomiting	no	
tonsillitis	**12(66,7%)**	**2(16,7%)**	**1(7,7%)**	**78(67,8%)**	
					93(58.9%)
	4(22,2%)	3(25,0%)	10(76,9%)	14(12,2%)	
chronic otitis media					31(19,6%)
goitre	0	2(16,7%)	1(7,7%)	3(2,6%)	6(3,8%)
laryngeal tumour	0	0	0	3(2,6%)	3(1,9%)
	0	0	0	1(0,9%)	1(0,6%)
purulent rhinorrhea					
pharyngeal tumour	0	0	0	1(0,9%)	1(0,6%)
	0	0	0	1(0,9%)	1(0,6%)
tympanic perforation					
cleft lip	0	1(8,3%)	0	3(2,6%)	4(2,5%)
mass	0	0	1(7,7%)	0	1(0,6%)
right laterocervical					
	1(5,6%)	0	0	0	1(0,6%)
vocal cord polyp					
mass	0	0	0	1(0,9%)	1(0,6%)
anterocervical					
adenoide vegetation	0	1(8,3%)	0	4(3,5%)	5(3,2%)
papillomatosis laryngee	1(5,6%)	0	0	0	1(0,6%)
seromucosal otitis	0	0	0	3(2,6%)	3(1,9%)
laryngeal web	0	1(8,3%)	0	0	1(0,6%)
lingual mass	0	0	0	1(0,9%)	1(0,6%)
septal derivation	0	0	0	2(1,7%)	2(1,3%)
	0	2(16,7%)	0	0	2(1,3%)
floor of the mouth cyst					
Total	18(100%)	12(100%)	13(100%)	115(100%)	158(100 %)

39.5% of PONV in the sample (17/43) occurred in patients operated on for

chronic otitis media. 54.8% (17/31) of patients operated on for chronic otitis

media had PONV postoperatively.

J <u>Risk factors studied :</u>

<u>Table XXXII:</u> **PONV distribution according to patient gender and prophylaxis.**

Gender		Group A N(%)	Group B N(%)	Total(100%)	
Male	NVPO	5 (33,3)	10 (66,7)	15	
	No	23 (57,5)	17 (42,5)	40	P= 0,137
	Total	28 (50,9)	27(49,1)	55	
Female	NVPO	**10 (35,7)**	**18 (64,3)**	**28**	
	No	41 (54,7)	34 (45,3)	75	**P=0,120**
	Total	51 (49,5)	52 (50,5)	103	

Male Chi-square^2 =3.311 ddl= 3P=0   .346 fisher's exact test p = 0.137 odds ratio = 0, 3764
Female chi2=3.915 ddl= 3P=0   .271 Fisher exact test p = 0.120 odds ratio = 0.4642

Of the **28** patients with PONV, **35.7%** had received the

Dexamethasone (Group A) versus **64.3%** who received nothing (Group B).

P = 0,120

<u>Table XXXIII:</u> **Distribution of the occurrence of PONV according to tobacco consumption and antiemetic prophylaxis.**

Tobacco	Group	A N(%)	Group B N(%)	Total (100%)
yes	NVPO	1 (20)	4 (80)	5
	No	3 (100)	0 (0)	3
	Total	4 (50)	4(50)	8
not	NVPO	**14 (36,8)**	**24 (63,2)**	**38**
	No	61 (54,5)	51 (45,5)	112
	Total	75 (50)	75 (50)	150

In **smokers, 25%** of patients **(%)** who received prophylaxis had PONV compared

to **100% (4/4) of smokers who** did not receive prophylaxis. Fisher's exact test

for smokers **P = 0.143**

In **non-smokers, 18.7%** of patients **(14/75)** who had received prophylaxis had

PONV compared to **32% (24/75) of non-smoking patients** who had not

received prophylaxis. Fisher's exact test for non-smokers **P = 0.09**

62.5% of patients who smoke had PONV, i.e. **5/8**

However, **25.33% of non-smoking patients** had PONV, i.e. **38/150.**

<u>Table XXXIV:</u> **Distribution of PONV according to ASA classification and antiemetic prophylaxis.**

ASA classification		Group A N(%)	Group B N(%)	Total	
ASA	1NVPO	**15 (39,5)**	**23 (61,5)**	38	P=0 ,094
No		60 (55,6)	48 (44,4)	100	Odds

Total	75 (51,4)	71 (48,6)	*ratio=0.5241*	
ASA 2 NVPO	0 (0)	4(100)	4	
No	3 (50)	3(50)	6	P= 0,2
Total	3(30)	7(70)	10	
ASA 3 NVPO	0(0)	1(100)	1	
No	1(100)	0(0)	1	P= 1
Total	1(50)	1(50)	2	

Among **ASA 1** patients, **26%** had PONV, **10.3%** in **group A** and **15.7%** in **group B**.

ASA 1 Fisher's exact test **p= 0.094**

Odds Ratio: 0.5241 95% confidence interval [0.2273; 1.1795].

P=0.2 (ASA2)

<u>Table XXXV:</u> PONV according to anaesthetic agents and antiemetic prophylaxis.

Anesthetic products		Group A N(%)	Group B N(%)	Total	
Ketamine	NVPO	9 (40,9)	13 (59,1)	22	
	No	24 (64,9)	13 (35,1)	37	P= 0,105
	Total	33 (55,9)	26 (44,1)	59	
propofol	NVPO	**6 (37,5)**	**10 (62,5)**	**16**	P= 0,384
	No	25 (54,3)	21 (45,7)	46	
	Total	31 (50)	31 (50)	62	
thiopental	NVPO	8(40)	12 (60)	20	
	No	22 (48,6)	25 (51,4)	47	P= 0,789
	Total	30 (44,8)	37 (55,2)	67	
fentanyl	NVPO	12(33,3)	24 (66,7)	36	Odd ratio= 0,4179
	No	47 (54,7)	39 (45,3)	86	P= 0,046
	Total	59 (48,4)	63 (51,6)	122	
celocurine	NVPO	7 (41,2)	10 (58,8)	17	
	No	20 (46,5)	23 (53,5)	43	P=0,779
	Total	27 (45)	33 (55)	60	
vecuronium	NVPO	6(24)	19(76)	25	Odd ratio= 0,2429
	No	20 (57,1)	15 (42,9)	35	P= 0,017
	Total	26 (43,3)	34 (56,7)	60	
halothane	NVPO	9(42,9)	12 (57,1)	21	
	No	36 (61,0)	23 (39)	59	P= 0,201
	Total	45 (56,2)	35 (43,8)	80	
isoflurane	NVPO	4(30,8)	9 (69,2)	13	
	No	9 (33,3)	18 (66,7)	27	
	Total	13 (32,5)	27 (67,5)	40	

Under *propofol,* **37.5%** of patients with PONV had received Dexamethasone (Group A) versus **62.5%** who had not (Group B). **40.9%** had PONV despite prophylaxis (Group A) versus 59.1% (Group B) using Ketamine.

Table XXXVI: Distribution of PONV according to duration of intervention and anti-emetic prophylaxis.

Duration of the intervention	Group A N(%)	Group B N(%)	Total
<30NVPO	5 (62,5)	3 (37,5)	8
No	25 (58,1)	18 (41,9)	43P=1
Total	30 (58,8)	21 (41,2)	51
30-59NVPO	**2 (16,7)**	**10 (83,3)**	**12** Oddratio=0
No	23 (48,9)	24 (51,1)	47 ,2138
Total	25 (42,4)	34 (57,6)	59P= 0,054
60-89NVPO	1 (50)	1 (50)	2
No	7 (87,5)	1 (12,5)	8P= 0,377
Total	8 (80)	2 (20)	10
90-119NVPO	2 (40)	3 (60)	5
No	4 (50)	4 (50)	8P
Total	6 (46,2)	7 (53,8)	13
>120NVPO	**5 (31,2)**	**11 (68,8)**	16
No	5 (55,6)	4 (44,6)	9 **P= 6,077**
Total	10 (40)	15 (60)	25

Of the **12** patients with a procedure time of **30** and **59 minutes** and PONV, **16.7%** had received Dexamethasone (Group A) compared to **83.3%** who had not (Group B). The difference was not significant (p= 0.054).

Of the **16** patients with a procedure time of **>120 minutes** and PONV, **31.2%** had received Dexamethasone (Group A) versus **68.8%** who had not (Group B).

Table XXXVII: Distribution of PONV according to surgeon's qualification

Discomfort	Medical specialist		CES		
	staff	Frequency(%)	staff	Frequency(%)	Total
NVPO	**36**	32,7	**7**	14,6	**43(27,2%)**
no	**74**	67,3	**41**	85,4	**115(72,8%)**
Total	110	100	48	100	158(100%)

Fisher's exact test **P=0.020**
Odds Ratio: 2.8326 95% confidence interval [1.111; 8.2282].

32.7% of patients operated on by specialist doctors had PONV
i.e. (36/110) against 14.6% of those operated by the ESCs, i.e. (7/48)

Table XXXVIII: Distribution of patients according to time of onset of <u>PONV</u> with or without antiemetic prophylaxis (n=43)

time slot of appearance	Group A Actual	Frequency(%)	Group B number	Frequency(%)	Total
between 0 and 6 hours post operative	**12**	85,7	**25**	86,4	**37(86%)**
between 7 and 12 hours post operative	**3**	14,3	**2**	9,1	**5(11,6%)**
between 19 and 24 hours post operative	**0**	0	**1**	4,5	**1(2,3%)**
Total	15	100	28	100	43(100%)

85.7% of patients in group A and **86.4%** in group B had **PONV** between **0 and 6 hours** after surgery.

The occurrence of PONV within the first 6 hours is **67.6%** in the absence of prophylaxis versus **32.4%** with prophylaxis.

Fisher's exact test p= 0.563

Table XXXIX: Distribution of PONV according to time of onset and food intake

Discomfort, time of onset / Food pick-up schedule		between 0 and 6 hours post-op	between 7 and 12 hours post-operatively	between 19 and 24 hours post-op	TOTAL
0 a 6ᵉ hours	NVPO	**25 (92,6%)**	**1 (3,7%)**	1(3,7%)	27
7ᵉ to 12e time	NVPO	11 (84,6%)	2(15,4%)	0	13
13th to 18th time	NVPO	1(33,3%)	2(66,7%)	0	3
	Total	37	5	1	43

25 patients had PONV between **0 and** $6i^{\otimes me}$ **hours** and these had resumed feeding between **0 and** $6i^{\otimes me}$ **hours.** These patients represent 58.1% of those with PONV.

Table XL: Postoperative patient progress.

	prognosis	
	death	Living
Patient progress		
total	0	158

No deaths were recorded during the course of the study.

VI COMMENTS AND DISCUSSION

1. Limitations of the methodology

The aim of our study was to evaluate the effect of dexamethasone in the prevention of PONV in patients undergoing surgery for ENT diseases.

The difficulties encountered in the course of this study were that :

> some patients were discharged less than 24 hours after surgery.

> Difficulty in sourcing dexamethasone 4mg ampoule.

> Postponement of scheduled procedures due to non-availability of anaesthetic products.

Given the paucity of work in Africa on PONV, we relied mainly on articles and studies in reputable journals in Europe, North America and Asia to compare our findings.

2. Incidence

In our study, the incidence of PONV was **27.22% (43/158)** or **35.4%** without prophylaxis and **19.0%** with prophylaxis.

2.1. Socio-epidemiological factors

2.1.1. Age

The 43 patients with PONV were under 60 years of age. This result is similar to that of **YANNICK [5]** who found 91.7% of cases in a study carried out in all the surgical departments of the same hospital. Nevertheless, **FOFANA [80]**, in a study of 232 patients, found that 71.2% of the subjects who vomited were under 60 years of age as opposed to 28.8% over 60 years of age [68], which makes it possible to affirm that ageing reduces the risk of PONV. This could be explained by the fact that younger subjects are more anxious about undergoing surgery compared to older ones.

2.1.2. Weight

The impact of weight, or more precisely body mass index (BMI), on the occurrence of PONV remains highly controversial. **WATCHA** is in favour **[23],**

KRANKE against **[61]**. In our study we found that 62.8% of patients with PONV weighed more than 60 kg. This supports the **SFAR** idea that weight overload is classically implicated as a factor in PONV.

2.1.3. Background

The main underlying conditions identified in our study were peptic ulcer and hypertension. The proportion of patients with a medical history was quite low in our study (**15.8%**).

2.1.4. risk factors

2.1.4.1.   Gender

In our study, 15 out of 55 men (**27.3%**) had PONV compared to **27.2%** of women (28/103) with a sex ratio of 1.87 in favour of the female sex. The incidence of PONV was almost identical in both sexes. The female sex does not influence the occurrence of PONV.

In the **28** patients with PONV, **35.7%** had received dexamethasone compared to **64.3%** who had not. Dexamethasone prophylaxis therefore reduced the risk of PONV in the female sex from **64.3%** to **35.7%**.

2.1.4.2.   Tobacco

Eight patients smoked, of whom **five** (62.**5%**) developed PONV. In contrast, the incidence of PONV in non-smokers was **25.33%** or **32%** in Group B, compared with **18.7%** in Group A. This equates to an odds ratio of **1.10** in the absence of prophylaxis versus 1.89 with antiepileptic prophylaxis.

SINCLAIR [51] found a PR of **1.4**, **APFEL** [61] a PR of **1.8**, both in the absence of prophylaxis. Thus we found no statistically significant relationship between PONV, antiemetic prophylaxis and non-smoking (p= 0.09). This is partly explained by the minority of smokers compared to non-smokers. In contrast, dexamethasone decreased the risk of PONV in non-smokers from **32%** to **18.7%**.

2.1.4.3. The ASA classification

92.4% (146/158) of the patients in our study were classified as ASA I, of which we found 38 cases of PONV or **26%** (38/146).

Dexamethasone decreased the risk of PONV in this group from **32.4%** to **20%**. The difference was not significant (p= 0.094)

2.1.4.4. APFEL score.

100 patients or 63.3% of our sample had 2 risk factors, 48 in Group A and 52 in Group B. The incidence of PONV was 19.0% and 35.4% respectively in each group.

2.1.4.5. Type of anaesthesia

All our patients were operated on under general anaesthesia with tracheal intubation.

2.2. Perioperative period

2.2.1. Anesthetic products

Thiopental was the most commonly used hypnotic in patients at 42.4% (67/158).

The occurrence of PONV was higher in patients who received **ketamine** as a hypnotic: 37.3% (22/59) compared to 29.8% (20/67) for **Thiopental**. This result confirms the superior emetic effect of ketamine compared to other hypnotics. However, there was no statistically significant difference (P= 0.789). Nevertheless, dexamethasone decreased the risk of PONV occurrence from 50% to 27.3% for Ketamine (p= 0.105).

Propofol, the product best indicated for its antiemetic properties, was administered to only 62 patients. **25.8%** of the patients on **propofol (16/62)** experienced PONV. Of these **37.5%** had received dexamethasone and the remaining **62.5%** had received nothing. In group A, **19.4%** of the patients (6/31) had PONV against **32.3%** of the patients in group B (10/31). Although the difference was not statistically significant, the risk of PONV was reduced by the use of prophylactic medication.

Of the **80** patients who received halothane, **21** or **26.2%** had PONV and of the 40 who received isoflurane **13** or **32.5%** had PONV. According to **APFEL**, halogen vapours are all potentially emetogenic **[39]**. Dexamethasone prophylaxis decreased the risk of PONV from **34.3%** to **20%** and **33.3% to 30.8%** (p=0.201 and p=) for halothane and isoflurane respectively.

2.2.2. Duration of the intervention

59 of our patients, i.e. **37.3%** (59/158), had an intervention time of between 30 and 59 minutes with an average time of 58.6 minutes. This is less than the study by **BASTIA et al** [26] which was **102 minutes.** Of these 59 patients, **20.3%** (12/59) had PONV. Dexamethasone reduced this risk from 83.3% to 16.7%, but the difference was not significant (p= 0.054).

In contrast, the incidence of PONV was higher in patients whose procedure duration was > 120 minutes, i.e. **64%** (16/25). This suggests that long procedures increase the risk of PONV; this is not statistically significant with a p=6.077

2.2.3. Post-operative analgesia

Paracetamol was the most commonly used postoperative analgesic. The 147 patients who were treated with injectable paracetamol had a PONV rate of **27.2%**. Noramidopyrine was administered in 6 patients; this was due to the low cost of the product. Acupan and paracetamol were combined in 2 patients. Morphine was not administered to any patient.

Post-operative period

2.2.4. The onset of PONV

Authors	Incidence of PONV without Prophylaxis	Incidence of PONV with Prophylaxis	p-value
APFEL, Canada, 2004 [49] N=5161	38,7%	28,5%	P< 0,001
WANG, 1999 [92] N= 90	63%	23%	P< 0,001
MAYEUR [93] N=395	39,2%	7,3%	P< 0,001
ODIN, 2004 [94] N= 109	24,5%	19,5%	P= 0,326
BENOIT, France, 2007 [95] N=	26%	9%	P< 0,001

860			
FOFANA A , 2011, N=232	52,6%	26,7%	P< 0,001
Our study N = 158	35,4%	19,0%	P=0,031

Our study found a total occurrence of PONV of **27.22% (43/158)** or **35.4%** in the absence of prophylaxis and **19.0%** with prophylaxis. **Anti-epileptic prophylaxis with Dexamethasone reduced the incidence of PONV from 35.4% to 19.0%. It therefore divided the risk of PONV occurrence and this difference was statistically significant with a p=0.031.** These figures are similar to those of **WANG** who found that dexamethasone prophylaxis reduced the risk of PONV from **63%** to **23% in patients undergoing laparoscopic cholecystectomy [73]. APFEL [36] found an incidence of 38.7% in the absence of prophylaxis, and 28.5% after prophylaxis with dexamethasone. BENOIT, in France, found a percentage of 26% of patients who suffered from PONV in the absence of prophylaxis against 9% after prophylaxis. MAYEUR for his part, in a study carried out on a sample of 395 patients, found a rate of 39.2% in the absence of prophylaxis, and 7.3% with prophylaxis. ODIN found 24.5% and 19.5% respectively in a study carried out in 2004 on 109 patients. FOFANA found 52.6% and 26.7% respectively in a study carried out in 2011 on 232 patients [80].**

2.2.5. Time of onset of discomfort

86% of the patients (37/43) had **PONV** between **0 and 6 hours** after surgery, i.e. **67.6%** in the absence of prophylaxis versus **32.4%** with dexamethasone prophylaxis. With p= 0.563 this difference was not significant but dexamethasone decreased the occurrence of PONV between 0 and 6 hours from 67.6% to 32.4%.

25 patients had PONV between **0 and 6ème hours** and these had resumed feeding between **0 and 6ième hours.** These patients represent 58.1% of those with PONV. This supports the idea that **early oral rehydration of** patients would favour the occurrence of PONV [56].

2.2.6. Antiemetic treatment

In our study, 13.9% of the patients, i.e. 6/43, received antiemetic treatment, i.e. 4 in Group A and 2 in Group B; these were patients who had experienced more than 2 episodes of vomiting after their awakening. Our patients received a monotherapy based on metopimazine (vogalene®) which is a dopamine antagonist 10 mg IM or IV every 12 hours.

2.3. Accidents

In our work, we have not observed any product-related accidents, where there is a high or medium risk of postoperative nausea and vomiting, a single prophylactic dose of dexamethasone is antiemetic, with no evidence of clinically significant toxicity [76].

CONCLUSION

Nausea and vomiting are important concerns and discomforts for patients in the postoperative period, although they are sometimes overlooked by nursing staff as they rarely have a fatal outcome. Our study shows that the incidence of PONV in ENT surgery is 27.2%. Chronic otitis media surgery is a major source of PONV despite the use of prophylactic medication. PONV in ENT surgery is mostly early onset, i.e. the first 6 hours. Thiopental was the most commonly used hypnotic. Ketamine induces a significant amount of PONV. Whatever the risk factor, dexamethasone prophylaxis reduced the occurrence of PONV. ENT surgery patients are a priori exposed to PONV, so our study allowed us to better evaluate the interest of antiemetic prophylaxis, particularly dexamethasone in ENT surgery at Gabriel Toure Hospital. Therefore, all surgical and anaesthetic staff should commit to the adoption of a dexamethasone prophylactic protocol aiming to reduce or even eradicate the incidence of PONV, even though many reviews state that the best PONV prophylaxis currently available is obtained by combining dexamethasone with a 5-HT3 receptor antagonist.

RECOMMENDATIONS

At the end of this study, we make the following suggestions:

1. To the administrative authorities

- To ensure that operating theatres and recovery rooms are adequately equipped to improve operating and recovery conditions;

- Ensure the availability and permanent accessibility of the most effective anti-emetic drugs, which are not available in our hospitals and pharmacies, for a better management of PONV.

- Provide ongoing training, supervision and refresher courses for health workers on the prevention and management of PONV

2. To the nursing staff of the ENT and anaesthesia department

- To promote a good collaboration between surgeons and anaesthetists in order to have a better follow-up of the patient from the pre-anaesthetic consultation to the hospital discharge;

- To be aware of the discomfort of patients with PONV and to prevent and manage it when it occurs.

Systematize the collection of the apfel score during pre-anaesthetic consultations.

- Add 8mg Dexamethasone to the operating kit of any patient with two or more risk factors according to the Apfel score.

- The systematic implementation by the anaesthesia team of a PONV prevention protocol according to the number of risk factors. -Psychological support for patients awaiting surgery so that they can approach their operation without anxiety or stress.

3. To patients.

-Keep calm and serenity before any operation;

-Notification of any previous cases of PONV at the pre-anaesthetic consultation.

REFERENCES

1. Pierre S. Nausea and postoperative vomiting. Unite fonctionnelle d'anesthesie reanimation, Institut Claudius Regaud, Toulouse. JMARU 2007.

2. Borgeat A. Nausea and postoperative vomiting. Conferences d'actualisation de la SFAR, Elsevier, Paris, 1996: p. 33-42.

3. Macario A, Weinger M, Carney S, Kim A. Which clinical anesthesia outcomes are important to avoid? The perspective of patients. Anesth Analg 1999; 89: 6528.

4. Benhamou D, Ribeyrolles D. Nausea and postoperative vomiting. In Nausea and postoperative vomiting (Monday 13 April 2009) CHU Bicetre Paris, France, www.ifits.fr.

5. Tala TY. Etude des Nausees et Vomissements Postoperatoires a l'Hopital Gabriel Toure de Bamako. These de Medecine, 2008; n°08M189.

6. Gan T, Sloan F, Dear G, El-moalem HE, Lubarsky DA. How much are patients willing to pay to avoid postoperative nausea and vomiting? Anesth Analg 2001; 92: 393-400.

7. Tramcr MR. A rational approach to the control of postoperative nausea and vomiting: evidence from systematic reviews. Part I. Efficacy and harm of antiemetic interventions, and methodological issues. Acta Scand Anaesthesiol 2001; 45: 4-13.

8. Palazzo MG, Strunin L. Anaesthesia and emesis. I: Etiology.
Can Anaesth Soc J 1984; **31**:178-87.

9. Palazzo M, Evans R. Logistic regression analysis of fixed patient factors for postoperative sickness: a model for risk assessment.*Br J Anaesth* 1993; **70**:13540

10. Apfel CC, Laara E, Koivuranta M, Greim CA, Roewer N. A simplified risk score for predicting postoperative nausea and vomiting: conclusions from crossvalidations between two centers. *Anesthesiology* 1999; **91**: 693-700.

11. Van Wijk MGF, Smalhout B. A postoperative analysis of the patient's view of anaesthesia in a Netherlands' teaching hospital. *Anaesthesia* 1990; **45**: 679-82.

12. **Hill RP, Lubarsky DA, Phillips-Bute B, et al.** Cost-effectiveness of prophylactic antiemetic therapy with ondansetron, droperidol or placebo. Anesthesiology 2000; 92: 958-7.

13. **Scuderi PE, James RL, Harris L, Mims GR 3rd.** Antiemetic prophylaxis does not improve outcomes after outpatient surgery when compared to symptomatic treatment. *Anesthesiology* ,1999; **90**: 360-71.

14. **G. Giguet, N. Bourdaud** Nausea and post-operative vomiting in adults and children. SFAR 2010 ; 22-25 September

15. **Borison HL, Wang SC.** Further Studies on the Vomiting Center. Federation Proceedings 1950; 9:14-15.

16. **Mannix KA.** Nausea and vomiting In: **Doyle D, Hanks GWC, MacDonald N.** Oxford textbook of palliative Medicine. Oxford University Press; 1998; 2nd edition.

17. **Goldberg SL.** The afferent paths of nerves involved in the vomiting reflex induced by distension of the isolated pyloric pouch. Am J Physiol 1931; 99:156159.

18. **Buttner MT.** Haloperidol in the prevention and treatment of nausea and vomiting: a systematic review of randomized controlled trials. **These de Medecine, Geneva, 2004;** No 10407: 8-20.

19. **De Medicis A.** Nausea and vomiting: physiopathology and therapeutic approach CHUM, 10 May 2002.

20. **Yuill G, Gwinnutt C.** Postoperative nausea and vomiting in World Federation of Societies of Anaesthesia (editors). **UPDATE IN ANAESTHESIA** , French version, ISSN 1353-4882, Year 2003; 17: 2-7.

21. **Naylor RJ, Inall FC.** The physiology and pharmacology of postoperative nausea and vomiting. Anaesthesia 1994; 49(Suppl):2-5

22. **SFAR 2007.** Management of postoperative nausea and vomiting;2 **23. Watcha MF, White PF.** Postoperative nausea and vomiting. Its etiology, treatment, and prevention. Anesthesiology 1992; 77:162-84.

24. **Faculte de Medecine U.L.P. de Strasbourg.** La surveillance de reveil post-anesthesique; 2003: 7.

25. **Koivuranta M, Laara E, Snare L, Alahuhta S.** A survey of postoperative nausea and vomiting. Aneasthesia 1997; 52: 443-9.

26. **Bastia B, Choquet O, Delchambre A, Gensollen S, Bongrand MC, Timon P, Manelli JC, Sambuc R.** Postoperative nausea and vomiting: analysis of risk factors. Pharmacie Hospitaliere Fran^aise 1999; 126: 45-48.

27. **Pierre S, Benais H, Pouymayou J.** Simplified Apfel scoring can favourably predict the risk of postoperative nausea and vomiting. Canadian Journal of Anesthesia 2002; 49:237-42.

28. **Gold BS, Kitz DS, Lecky JH, Neuhaus JM.** Unanticipated admission to the hospital following ambulatory surgery. JAMA 1989; 262: 3008-10.

29. **Tramer MR, Moore A, McQuay H.** Prevention of vomiting after paediatric strabismus surgery: a systematic review using the numbers-needed-to-treat method. Br J Anaesth 1995; 75: 556-61.

30. **Van Den Berg A, Lambourne A, Clyburm PA.** The oculoemetic reflex. A rationalisation of postophthalmic anaesthesia vomiting. Anaesthesia 1989; 44:100-7.

31. **Haigh CG, Kaplan LA, Durham JM, Dupeyron JP, Harmer M, Kenny GN.** Nausea and vomiting after gynaecological surgery: a meta-analysis of factors affecting their incidence. Br J Anaesth 1993; 71: 517-22.

32. **Gratz I, Allen E, Afshar M, Joslyn AF, Buxbaum J, Prilliman B.** The effects of the menstrual cycle on the incidence o emesis and efficacy of ondansetron. Anesth Analg 1996; 83: 565-9.

33. **Saiah M, Borgeat A, Tramer M, Rifat K.** Does the surgical technique

influence the incidence of postoperative nausea/vomiting after strabismus surgery in children? Br J Anaesth 1995; 74 (Suppl 1): 99.

34. **Cohen MM, Duncan PG, De Boer DP, Tweed WA.** The post-operative interview: assessing risk factors for nausea and vomiting. Anesth Analg 1994; 78: 7-16.

35. **Andersen R, Krogh K.** Pain as a major cause of postoperative nausea. Can Anaesth Soc J 1976; 23: 366-9.

36. **Salmenpera M, Kuoppamaki R, Salmenpera A.** Do anti-cholinergic agents affect the occurrence of postanaesthetic nausea? Acta Anaesthesiol Scand 1992; 36: 445-8.

37. **Ratra CK, Badola RP, Bhargava KR.** A Study of factors concerned in emesis during spinal anaesthesia. Br J Anaesth 1972; 44:1208-11.

38. **Carpenter RL, Caplan RA, Brown DL, Stephenson C, WU R.** Incidence and risk factors for side effects of spinal anesthesia. Anesthesiology 1992; 76: 906-16.

39. **Pusch F, Freitag H, Weinstabl C, Obwegeser R, Huber R, Widling E.** Singleinjection paravertebral block compared to general anaesthesia in breast surgery. Acta Anaesthesiol Scand 1999; 43: 770-4.

40. **Apfel CC, Korttila K, Abdalla M, Kerger H, Turan A, Vedder I, et al**. A factorial trial of six interventions for the prevention of postoperative nausea and vomiting. N Engl J Med 2004; 350: 2441-51.

41. **Raferty S, Sherry E.** Total intravenous anaesthesia with propofol and alfentanil protects against postoperative nausea and vomiting. Can J Anaesth 1991; 39:37-40.

42. **Gunawardene RD, White DC.** Propofol and emesis. Anaesthesia 1988; 43 (Suppl):65-7.

43. **Korttila K, Ostman P, Faure E, Apfelbaum JL, Prunskis J, Ekdawi M.** Randomized comparison of recovery after propofol-nitrous oxide versus

thiopentone-isoflurane-nitrous oxide anaesthesia in patients undergoing ambulatory surgery. Acta Anaesthesiol Scand 1990; 34:400-3.

44. Perreault L, Normandin N, Plamondon L, Blain R, Rousseau P, Girard M. Middle ear pressure variations during nitrous oxide and oxygen anaesthesia. Can Anaesth Soc J 1982; 29: 428-34.

45. Melnick BM, Johnson LD. Effects of eliminating nitrous oxide in outpatient anesthesia. Anesthesiology 1987; 67:982-4.

46. Apfel CC, Katz MH, Kranke P, Goepfert C, Papenfuss T, Rauch S. Volatile anaesthesia may be the main cause of early but not delayed postoperative vomiting: a randomized controlled trial of factorial design. Br J Anaesth 2002; 88: 1-10.

47. Hovorka J, Korttila K, Erkola O. Nitrous oxide does not increase nausea and vomiting following gynaecological laparoscopy. Can J Anaesth 1989; 36:145-8.

48. Hovorka J, Kortilla K, Erkola O. The experience of the person ventilating the lungs does influence postoperative nausea and vomiting. Acta Anaesthesiol Scand 1990; 34: 203-589.

49. Janhunen L, Tammisto T. Postoperative vomiting after different modes of general anaesthesia. Ann Chir Gynaecol Fenniae 1972; 61:152-9.

50. Hovorka J, Korttila K, Erkola O. Gastric aspiration at the end of anaesthesia does not decrease postoperative nausea and vomiting. Anaesth Intensive Care 1990; 18: 58-61.

51. Cheatham ML, Chapman WC, Key SP, Sawyers JL. A meta-analysis of selective versus routine nasogastric decompression after elective laparotomy. Ann Surg 1993; 221: 469-76.

52. King MJ, Milazkiewicz R, Carli F, Deacock AR. Influence of neostigmine on postoperative vomiting. Br J Anaesth 1988; 61: 403-6.

53. Andersen R, Krohg K. Pain as a major cause of postoperative nausea. Can Anaesth Soc J 1976; 23: 366-9.

54. **Jakobsson J, Davidson S, Andreen M, Westgreen M.** Opioid supplementation to propofol anaesthesia for outpatient abortion: a comparison between alfentanil, fentanyl and placebo. Acta Anaesthesiol Scand 1991; 35: 767-70.

55. **Parnass SM, McCarthy RJ, Ivankovich AD.** The role of pain as a cause of postoperative nausea/vomiting after outpatient anesthesia. Anesth Analg 1992; 74:S 233.

56. **Yogendran S, Asokumar B, Cheng DC, Chung F.** A prospective randomized double-blinded study of the effect of intravenous fluid therapy on adverse outcomes on outpatient surgery. Anesth Analg 1995; 80: 682-6.

57. **Hechler A, Naujoks F, Ataman K, Hopf HB.** Die Inzidenz an postoperativer Ubelkeit und Erbrechen ist unahangig von der routinema^igen Maskenvorbeatmung wahrend der Narkoseeinleitung. Anasthesiol Intensivmed Notfallmed Schmerzther 1999; 34: 684-8.

58. **Jin F, Norris A, Chung F, Ganeshram T.** Should adult patients drink fluids before discharge from ambulatory surgery? Anesth Analg 1998; 87: 306-11

59. **Sinclair DR, Chung F, Mezei G.** Can postoperative nausea and vomiting be predicted? Anesthesiology 1999; 91: 109-18.

60. **Apfel CC, Laara E, Koivuranta M, Greim CA, Roewer N.** A simplified risk score for predicting postoperative nausea and vomiting: conclusions from crossvalidations between two centers. Anesthesiology 1999; 91: 693-700.

61. **Badaoui R, Pouilly A, Yagoubi A, Carpentier F, Riboulot M, Ossart M.** Comparison of the efficacy of ondansetron and droperidol in the prevention of postoperative nausea and vomiting. Cahier d'Anesthesiologie 1999; 47: 297-301.

62. **Palazzo M, Evans R.** Logistic regression analysis of fixed patient factors for postoperative sickness: a model for risk assessment. Br J Anaesth 1993; 70:13540.

63. **Honkavaara P, Lehtinen AM, Hovorka J, Korttila K.** Nausea and vomiting after gynaecological laparoscopy depends upon the phase of the menstrual cycle. Can J Anaesth 1991; 38: 876-9.

64. **Beattie W, Lindblad T, Buckley D, Forrest J.** Menstruation increases the risk of nausea and vomiting after laparoscopy. A prospective randomized study. Anesthesiology 1993; 78: 272-6.

65. **Ramsay TM, McDonald PF, Faragher EB.** The menstrual cycle and nausea or vomiting after wisdom teeth extraction. Can J Anaesth 1994; 41: 798-80.

66. **Saeeda I, Jain PN**. Post-operative nausea and vomiting (PONV): A review article. Indian J. Anaesth 2004; 48 (4): 253-258.

67. **Sweeney BP.** Why does smoking protect against PONV? Br J Anaesth 2002; 89: 810-3.

68. **Toner CC, Broomhead CJ, Littlejohn JH, Samra GS, Pwner JG, Palazzo MG.** Prediction of postoperative nausea and vomiting using a logistic regression model. Br J Anaesth 1996; 76: 347-51.

69. **Junger A, Hartmann B, Benson M, Schindler E, Dietrich G, Jost A.** The use of an anesthesia information management system for prediction of antiemetic rescue treatment at the postanesthesia care unit. Anesth Analg 2001; 92: 1203.

70. **Apfel CC, Kranke P, Eberhart LH, Roos A, Roewer N.** Comparison of predictive models for postoperative nausea and vomiting. Br J Anaesth 2002; 88: 234-40.

71. **Domino KB, Anderson EA, Polissar NL, Posner KL.** Comparative efficacy and safety of ondansetron, droperidol and metoclopramide for preventing postoperative nausea and vomiting: a meta-analysis. Anesth Analg 1999; 88: 1370-9.

72. **P.Diemunsch** management of postoperative nausea and vomiting. Conference of experts - short text, SFAR congress September 2007.

73. **Tramer MR.** Rational control of PONV - the rule of three. Can J Anesth

2004; 51: 283-5.

74. Bolton CM, Myles PS, Nolan T, Sterne JA. Prophylaxis of postoperative vomiting in children undergoing tonsillectomy: a systematic review and metaanalysis. Br J Anaesth 2006;97:593-604

75. Henzi I, Walder B, Tramer MR. Dexamethasone for the prevention of nausea and vomiting: a quantitative systematic review. Anesth Analg 2000; 90:186-94

76. Sfar 2008. Postoperative nausea and vomiting

77. Kim MS, Cote CJ, Cristoloveanu C et al There is no dose-escalation response to dexametha- sone (0.0625-1.0 mg/kg) in pediatric tonsillectomy or adenotonsillectomy patients for preventing vomiting , reducing pain, shortening time to first liquid int ake, or the incidence of voice change. Anesth Analg 20 07;104:1052-8

78. Wang JJ, Ho ST, Tzeng JI, Tang CS. The effect of timing of dexamethasone administration on its efficacy as a prophylactic antiemetic for postoperative nausea and vomiting. Anesth Analg 2000; 91:136-9

79. corticoide [online]. [cited 03 July 2014].available: http:/ / en. wikipedia. org/ w/ index. php?title=Cortico%C3%AFde& action=edit

80. FOFANA A. Interet de la dexamethasone dans la prevention des nausees et vomissements post operatoires en chirurgie viscerale [my thesis:Med]. Bamako : University of Bamako ; 2011 : p 84

Annex 1
Survey and data collection form

Sheet No. :

date :

		20

I. **Socio-demographic data**

Q1. <u>Name and surname</u> :

Q2. Age: Q3. <u>Weight:</u>Q4. <u>Sex:</u> Male: 1 Female: 2

Q5. <u>Profession:</u> Civil servant:1 Tradesman/Salesperson:2
Student:3 Farmer:4 Driver:5 Military:6
Housewife: 7 Unemployed: 8
 Bamako: 1 Interior: 2

Q6. <u>Place of residence</u> :

II. **Background (personal)**

Q7. <u>Medical history</u> :
1. Gastro resophageal reflux
2. Gastro duodenal ulcer
3. Postoperative nausea and vomiting
4. Diabetes
5. Arterial hypertension
6. Tuberculosis
7. Travel sickness
8. Anxiety
9. Asthma
10. Other   yes: 1 no: 2
11. No history
if yes, please specify:
Q8. <u>Surgical history</u> :

1. Number of previous surgeries
2. Indications/diagnosis:

Q9. Obstetrical <u>and gynecological history</u> :

Gestite Parite Abortion Decedent children Living children

Is she pregnant? If so, which trimester?

Q10. <u>Lifestyle</u> :

1. Tobacco: if yes, number of packs/years
2. Alcohol :

3. Cafe :

4. The :

Other details :

5. No special features:

111.   The pre-operative patient

Q11 <u>Time between last meal and surgery</u>:

1. less than 12 hours

2. between 12 and 18 hours

3. between 18:00 and 24:00

4. beyond 24 hours

Q12 <u>Premedication administered</u> :

5. Diazepam

6. Atropine

7. Morphine

8. Other   specify :

9. Not done

Q13 <u>Patient classification by ASA</u>: ASA

IV. <u>The intraoperative patient</u>

Q14. <u>planned surgery</u>: _ yes: 1 no: 2

Q15. <u>operating technique</u> :

Q16 <u>Intraoperative diagnosis</u> :

Q17. <u>Qualification of the surgeon</u>: Specialist:1 ESC:2 Generalist: 3

Q18 <u>Qualification of the anaesthetist</u>:| Physician: 1 Medical assistant: 2

DES: 3

Q19. <u>type of anaesthesia</u>

general: 1 local-regional: 2

Q20. <u>Anaesthetic products used (induction, maintenance)</u> :

1. Ketamine
2. Propofol
3. Bupivacaine
4. Thiopental
5. Fentanyl
6. Fluothane
7. Celocurine
8. Marcaine
9. Nitrous oxide
10. Penthotal
11. Xylocaine
12. Vecuronium
13. Dexamethasone
Other if yes, please specify:
Q21. Intubation: orotracheal: 1 nasotracheal: 2 not done: 3
Q22 Nasogastric tube :
perop: 16 hours postop: 2
Q23. Antiemetic prophylaxis: yes: 1 no: 2

Q24. Scope: yes: 1 no: 2
Q25. Blood transfusion: yes: 1 no: 2
Q26. Duration of the intervention
hour(s) minutes

. **The postoperative patient**
Q26. Duration of the intervention

Q27. Postoperative analgesia :
1. Tramadol
2. Noramidopyrin
3. Morphine
4. Ibuprofen
5. Ketoprofene
6. Paracetamol
7. Other   if
Q28. Decurarisation: Neostigmine: 1 Atropine: 2
other: 3, to be specified: not done: 4
Q29. Apfel score :
Q30. type of discomfort: nausea: 1 vomiting: 2
nausea and vomiting: 3 none: 4

Q31. If discomfort, specify the time of onset:

Between 0 and 6 hours postoperatively: 1
Between 7 and 12 hours postoperatively: 2
Between 13 and 18 hours postoperatively: 3
Between 19 and 24 hours postoperatively: 4
Between 25 and 48 hours postoperatively: 5
Q32. If vomiting, specify appearance:
Liquid: 1
Food: 2
Hematic (reddish): 3
Bilious (greenish or yellowish): 4
Fecaloid: 5
Q33. If discomfort, specify duration: hours
Q34. If PONV, complications :
Mendelson syndrome (bronchial inhalation): 1
Mallory-Weiss syndrome (heart ulceration): 2
Suture laches: 3
Burns (L'sopliagieinies: 4
Metabolic alkalosis: 5
Other: 6 to be specified :
No complications: 7
Q35. If PONV, anti-emetic treatment administered: yes: 1 no: 2

If yes, please specify which one:
Q36. Side effects : yes: 1 no: 2 if yes, specify:
th postoperative hour. no: 2

Q38. Patient satisfaction: yes: 1
If so, why?
If not, why not?

<u>**APPENDIX 2:**</u> American Society of Anesthesiologists (ASA) classification of patient clinical status

ASA 1	Normal or healthy patient
ASA 2	Patient with a mild systemic disease
ASA 3	Patient with a serious systemic condition, which limits activity without causing disability
ASA 4	Patient with a disabling and life-threatening systemic condition
ASA 5	Moribund patients with a life expectancy of less than 24 hours, with or without intervention
ASA U	Emergency surgery patient

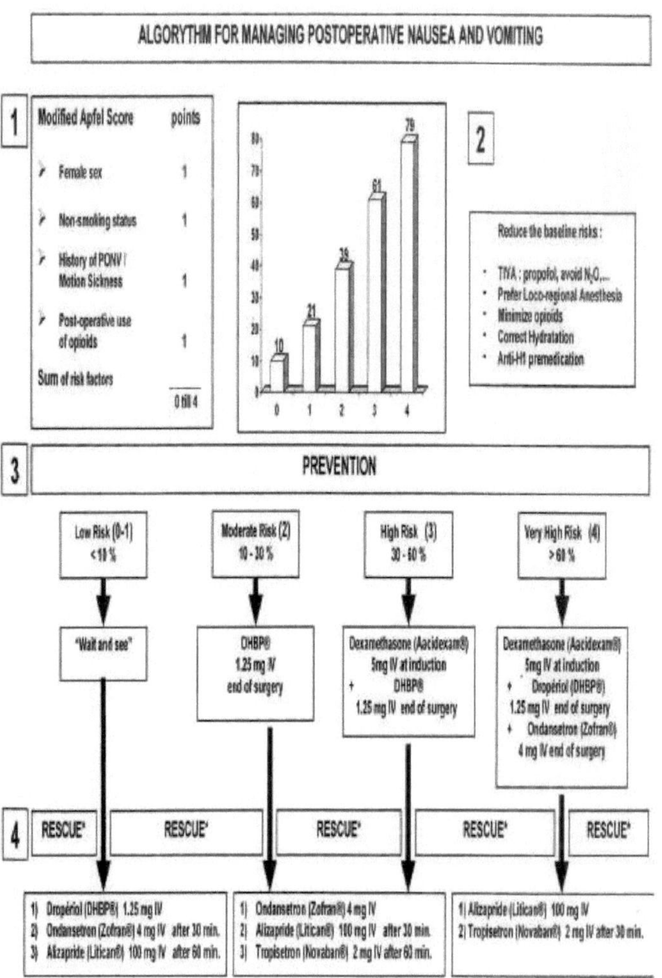
ALGORYTHM FOR MANAGING POSTOPERATIVE NAUSEA AND VOMITING

1
Modified Apfel Score   points

Female sex   1

Non-smoking status   1

History of PONV /
Motion Sickness   1

Post-operative use
of opioids   1

Sum of risk factors
0 till 4

2
Reduce the baseline risks :

TIVA : propofol, avoid N₂O,...
Prefer Loco-regional Anesthesia
Minimize opioids
Correct Hydratation
Anti-H1 premedication

3   PREVENTION

Low Risk (0-1)
< 10 %

Moderate Risk (2)
10 - 30 %

High Risk (3)
30 - 60 %

Very High Risk (4)
> 60 %

"Wait and see"

DHBP®
1.25 mg IV
end of surgery

Dexamethasone (Aacidexam®)
5mg IV at induction
+
DHBP®
1.25 mg IV end of surgery

Dexamethasone (Aacidexam®)
5mg IV at induction
+   Dropériol (DHBP®)
1.25 mg IV end of surgery
+   Ondansetron (Zofran®)
4 mg IV end of surgery

4   RESCUE*   RESCUE*   RESCUE*   RESCUE*   RESCUE*

1) Dropériol (DHBP®) 1.25 mg IV
2) Ondansetron (Zofran®) 4 mg IV after 30 min.
3) Alizapride (Liticar®) 100 mg IV after 60 min.

1) Ondansetron (Zofran®) 4 mg IV
2) Alizapride (Liticar®) 100 mg IV after 30 min.
3) Tropisetron (Novaban®) 2 mg IV after 60 min.

1) Alizapride (Liticar®) 100 mg IV
2) Tropisetron (Novaban®) 2 mg IV after 30 min.

*If problems occur within 6 hours post surgery, go to RESCUE (4) ; If problems occur after 6 hours post surgery : repeat prophylaxis (3)

Names: AGHOAGNI GOUAJIO

Prenoms : Gilles Gaël **e-mail :** agillesgael@yahoo.fr **Title of the thesis :** *Int£r6t de la Dexamëthasone dans la prevention des Nausees et Vomissements Postopëratoires en chirurgie ORL au Centre Hospitalier Universitaire Gabriel Touƶë de Bamako*

Academic year: 2013-2014

Location of the event: Bamako

Country of origin: CAMEROON

Place of deposit: Library of the Faculty of Medicine and Odontostomatology (FMOS) of Bamako.

Centre of interest: Anesthesia-Reanimation Department, ENT Department.

SUMMARY

Background: From November 2013 to May 2014, we conducted a randomised, single-blind study on the benefit of dexamethasone prophylaxis in the occurrence of postoperative nausea and vomiting in ENT surgery at the Gabriel Toure University Hospital in Bamako. This study was based on the analysis of pre-anesthetic consultations, anaesthesia records, post-operative treatment records and patient interviews.

Aims: The aim was to study the value of Dexamethasone in the prevention of PONV, through the description of the characteristics of PONV, the determination of the risk of its occurrence, and the analysis of its risk factors in relation to prophylaxis with Dexamethasone.

Results: A total of 158 patients were enrolled; 43 patients had PONV for an overall incidence of 27.22%; of which 35.4% (28/79) were without prophylaxis **(Group B)** versus 19.0% (15/79) with Dexamethasone prophylaxis **(Group A).**

The average age of the patients was 21.96 ± 15.40 years. Females were the most common sex in 65.2% of cases. Eight patients were smokers (5.1%). 92.4% of the patients were classified as ASA 1. 100 patients (63.3%) had 2 risk factors. 60.1% of the patients had received premedication; the most commonly used combination was diazepam and atropine in 49 patients. All procedures were performed under general anaesthesia with tracheal intubation. Thiopental was the most commonly used hypnotic with 42.4% or 38% (30/79) in group A and 46.8% (37/79) in group B. 37.3% of the patients had an intervention time between 30 and 59 minutes. The most common pathology operated on in the ENT surgery block was tonsillitis in 58.9% of cases with a PONV occurrence of 16.1%. On the other hand, 54.8% (17/31) of the patients operated on for chronic otitis media had PONV. 86% of patients (37/43) experienced discomfort between 0 and 6^e hours after surgery. Paracetamol was the most commonly used postoperative analgesic in 93% of cases.

Conclusion: ENT surgery is one of the surgeries in which the incidence of PONV remains high. Our study has therefore allowed us to better understand the value of antiemetic prophylaxis, particularly dexamethasone. As a result, all surgical and anaesthetic staff should commit to the adoption of a dexamethasone prophylaxis protocol in order to reduce or even eradicate the incidence of PONV. This will result in greater comfort for the patient and better management.

Keywords: PONV, prophylaxis, dexamethasone, risk of occurrence, incidence.

Name: AGHOAGNI GOUAJIO
First Name : Gilles Gaël
e-mail: agillesgael@yahoo.fr
Title of the thesis: Interest of the use of dexamethasone in the post operative prevention of nausea and vomiting in the ORL unit of the teaching hospital of Gabriel Toure in Bamako.
Academic year: 2013-2014
Place of the thesis: Bamako
Country of chargeability: Cameroon
Place of deposit: Health science's library of Bamako
Center of interest: unit of anesthesia and reanimation, unit of ORL

HIPPOCRATIC OATH

In the presence of the masters of this faculty, of my dear fellow students, before the effigy of Hippocrates, I swear in the name of the supreme being to be faithful to the laws of honour and probity in the practice of medicine.

I will give my free care to the needy and will never demand a salary above my work, I will not participate in any clandestine sharing of fees. My eyes shall not see what goes on inside the houses, my tongue shall not speak of the secrets entrusted to me, and my state shall not be used to corrupt errors or to promote crime.

I will not allow considerations of religion, nation, race, party or class to come between my duty and my patient. I will maintain absolute respect for human life from conception.

Even under threat, I will not allow my medical knowledge to be used against the laws of humanity.

Respectful and grateful to my teachers, I will give back to their children the education I received from their father.

May men esteem me if I am faithful to my promises. May I be shamed and despised by my colleagues if I fail to do so.

I swear it.